More Praise for *This Is Remission*

"I met Ryan in 2007 working on his album and we hit it off immediately. I got such joy working with someone who is such a fighter. Ryan time and again overcame health issues that many people give in to and showed such a drive to do what it took to make his record great. His songs really spoke to and inspired me, as they have to many people, and showed a real talent for songwriting. The future is wide open for Ryan, as he does not know the word quit, and I am proud to have been a small part of his musical life. Here is to continued success for the book Ryan, you rock!"

**—Jeff Tomei, Rockit Productions, Inc.,
jefftomeirockit.com**

"We are regularly inspired by the strength and courage with which our cancer patients respond to their undeserved adversities. Ryan's story is remarkably unique for its duration and success over multiple disease recurrences, for his ongoing strength to deal with the array of challenges caused by treatment-related toxicities (all too common in long term survivors), and now for his willingness and ability to share his story. Ryan's gift to us is profoundly life-affirming. He is one special person and an inspiration to us all."

—Jessica Neely, PA-C and Elliott Winton, M.D.

"Ryan's story is one of not just surviving, but also THRIVING, and he tells it with such honesty and humor. His Mom chimes in with her perspective. Having lost my 5 1/2 yo son, Aidan, to leukemia, I can really relate to her words. This book is a MUST READ for anyone who needs inspiration to overcome any challenge in life, but especially a life-threatening illness like cancer."

—Regina ("Regi") Garvey,
Advocate for raising funds for cancer research
in memory of her son, Aidan

"Ryan's story of survival is amazing. The last chapter of this book nails what it takes to get through tough times."

—John Walker, former U.S. Navy Seal,
Founder of Juice Alive

THIS IS REMISSION

A Four-Time Cancer Survivor's Memories of Treatment, Struggle, and Life

This Is Remission - A Four-Time Cancer Survivor's Memories of Treatment, Struggle, and Life

Copyright © 2019 Ryan Hamner

Book design by:
Arbor Services, Inc.
www.arborservices.co/

Printed in the United States of America

This Is Remission - A Four-Time Cancer Survivor's Memories of Treatment, Struggle, and Life
Ryan Hamner

1. Title 2. Author 3. Self-Help

Library of Congress Control Number: 2019901430
ISBN 13: 9781795661294

THIS IS REMISSION

A Four-Time Cancer
Survivor's Memories of
Treatment, Struggle, and Life

RYAN HAMNER

Contents

Introduction

Everything you've ever wanted is on the other side of fear.

– George Addair

Lying in the ER, the smells of bleach from the freshly cleaned floor and alcohol swirling over me, I was freezing even though buried deep in my sheets. I heard the nurse come into the room through the sliding door—*shhlink*—but I was looking behind me at the heart monitor above the bed. I could feel my heart going out of rhythm and my heart rate increasing, so you can bet my eyes were pinned to what the monitor showed me second by second.

While my nurse stood in front of the little red box on the wall full of dirty needles, I told her that something was happening with my heart. She assured me that I was in a regular rhythm and that everything was just fine. I could feel something off with my heart, but she was clearly telling me I was fine. Go figure? I guess I might have been pissed if I hadn't been so scared about feeling my heart acting so weird.

Then she asked: "Did you feel that?" She checked the name on my registration bracelet while looking up at the heart monitor. I practically shouted: "Yes!" feeling jolts and skipped beats come rapid-fire through my chest.

Um, I told you something was happening here, lady!

Within a few minutes, my heart rate and blood pressure were soaring. If I had been in a panic a minute earlier, I was now at DEFCON 5. My chest was pounding, alarms on my monitor sounded, and the medical staff rushed into my room. One nurse grabbed my left arm and another grabbed my right, trying to control my arms as they shook back and forth. These nurses were searching for veins—already damaged by chemotherapy—sturdy enough for the insertion of an IV needle. Boy, was this turning out to be a fun afternoon.

Eventually, after a few swabs with alcohol pads and a couple of sharp sticks, both nurses got an IV started. From here on in, I had a hard time keeping track of what was going on. Doctors were discussing what to do, rushing in and out of my room, either barking orders or talking and listening intently over their phones. As the oxygen cannula was being placed around my nose, the cardiologist on call rushed into the room, stared at my heart monitor, and then everyone looked at each other.

It was you-know-what hitting the fan; they knew it, and I knew that they knew I knew it. *Good*, I thought, best I could form a thought right then... *can we get on with keeping me from dying here, please?*

Soon, all the conversations and alarms were seeping into my brain as one muffled sound: chaos in the room, chaos in my head. Several people were coaching me to take slow, deep breaths through my nose, while my arms and legs continued to shake out of control. In a quick moment, however, it came, what we all knew was coming: my heart rate hit 250 beats per minute.

The cardiologist shouted: "We have to do something, now!"

Yeah, no kidding, dude.

A couple of nurses rushed out of my room, then came running back in and pushed meds through my IV. They had to do this slowly, though, for the meds to work, so it felt like a lifetime waiting (hoping) that whatever they were giving me would have some effect. As the nurses pushed the syringe and everyone in the room continued to study the heart monitor, the cardiologist pulled out a notepad, made a few notes, and glanced back at the monitor; the heart monitor's little screen was the focal point for us all. We were all waiting for my heart rate to start decreasing as the medicine was pushed through my IV.

My heart rate finally dropped to around 120 beats per minute, and everybody in the room breathed a big sigh of relief… nobody more than me, though. The medicine had worked.

I would spend the next two days in the ICU. I had survived, again.

Have you ever survived something incredible? Something that, looking back now, seems so surreal you have to ask yourself: "How did I do that?" and "Did I actually do that?"—an event that permanently changed you, made you stronger and wiser, gave you depth, but also ended up challenging you for the rest of your life?

Well, for me, the challenge was cancer. Surviving cancer four times took me on a journey that I would never have chosen at the time, but also a journey I'd never change now. It's kind of like studying martial arts, something I have spent a good chunk of time doing in my life. Yeah, it's a weird analogy, I know, but I'll make plenty of them in this book, so stick with me.

Putting in the hard work required to grow in any martial art isn't easy, and not everyone is up to applying the discipline required. However, many men and women who embark on this kind of mind-body-heart study do so because they genuinely want to master the craft and come to enjoy the "art" of the specific moves and the philosophy they come to learn. But to grow, martial artists must step outside of their comfort zones. They absolutely must be willing to make sacrifices and to take risks. They must endure pain, breaks, losses, disappointments, and healing.

Without the pain, losses, disappointments, and stepping outside of your comfort zone, growth will never come for any of us... in martial arts and in life. Wouldn't you agree? Without getting outside of what we know, what is habit, what we do so well it's second nature to us, we'll never live to the fullest. And sometimes stepping outside of that comfort zone, our routine, even to the side of our skills, is not a choice, like pushing yourself in a dōjō. Sometimes, that stepping far and wide—being uncomfortable in all manner of ways, and in ways that might hurt you or even come close to getting you killed—comes from a strong push that you might not have ever wanted or even seen coming.

But still, you are pushed beyond what you feel is your limit, like martial artists often push themselves. I was pushed often beyond any limit I ever thought I had, well beyond my comfort zone. And it was painful, scary, and life threatening, but because of cancer I endured and survived; I grew in ways I never could have otherwise. This book is not about a poor kid taking on cancer four times and his tale of woe. It's not about all the treatments that left me incapable of achieving my goals. I'd like to think this book is about the total opposite. I'd like to think the theme here is taking on cancer four times, beating it, and battling all the challenges it threw my way, with the help of some great people. Sometimes I cried, sometimes I almost died (sometimes I could rhyme... sorry, but I set myself up for that, so I had to use it), and sometimes I stood in abject fear of where I found myself and what might be coming next. But I stepped far left and right of my comfort zone and survived.

I've had many great opportunities, from writing books for children with cancer, to touring the country playing my music, and recording that music for my record deal, to becoming an avid martial artist, to befriending many courageous people along the way, to living my life and being loved by a wonderful family. I have heard it said that what doesn't kill you makes you stronger. I am living proof that what did not kill me has undoubtedly left me weaker in some physical respects, and occasionally maybe a little ill-equipped emotionally than I want to be, but never beaten as far as my spirit is concerned. Yes, my story will reveal my individual journey with cancer (and its cure), but I will also tell about my personal view of survivorship and how it is so different these days (thank God) than it was way back when I was first diagnosed.

And you won't hear only from me here. I will bring my dear not-so-old mom into the story to give you firsthand accounts when appropriate. As I will tell you time and again in this book, one of the most tragic long-lasting symptoms from all I have gone through is my terrible memory loss. That was the reason I often went to my mom when writing this story to help me recall someone's name or to have her piece together the chronological progression of events I had long since lost in my brain. And seeing as she was there from the beginning — when I first was diagnosed at age six — and stayed by my side all throughout my life with cancer, until my last round of treatment that ended with a transplant when I was twenty-one, and she is someone I adore above and beyond anyone else on this earth, why not have my mother chime in from time to time? Her perspective, as parent and caregiver, is so significant, I feel. She also figures into the last chapter, the one on survivorship, to give a firsthand account of what it is like for those wonderful caregivers we have who see us through to good health (and to inspire those who don't see their patients and loved ones to good health) and how she has come to see the future, as well as our now.

This is my story, for good or bad, healthy and sick, fun and ter-rible, but certainly truthful. I hope I bring some lightness into your day and that you will know me a little better after you read this book. For those of you who are presently undergoing treatment for cancer, I hope you get through as quickly as you can with as few side effects as possible. For those, like me, who are survivors, I am sure much of what I relate here will be all too familiar, and maybe at other times you will come to think, "No, Ryan, that's not how that happened for me," which is perfectly reasonable. Cancer, like many things in life, is unique to us all even if we have suffered the same diagnosis and treatments. For the caregiver, I hope you find something here to comfort you while you spend your days and so many of your sleepless nights worrying about the patient you are attending and love. And for those who have been lucky enough to have never had cancer come into your life, I hope by reading what I have written here, you will realize how blessed you are.

I wish every one of you the very best of health.

Now, on with the Ryan show.

Chapter 1

On Being a Ninja, Yo-Yo Spit, and Skinny Willie

There was never a night or a problem that could defeat sunrise or hope.

–Bernard Williams

Everyone has a different experience growing up. Even siblings living their childhood right next to one another, under the same roof, with the same parents experience life in their unique way. Nature and nurture—a sprinkling of both makes us who we are. Unique, wacky, flawed, wonderful human beings are what you get when we hit the ground running.

Now, some of us realize that our childhood was about the best anybody could have ever wished. With the benefit of hindsight, others of us come to realize that we lived in a wildly dysfunctional household, though it seemed normal at the time.

Hey, what did we know, right? And some of us never truly grow up; we grow older, yes, but never fully outgrow the childhood wonder of finding simple pleasure in things. Many times I have considered this option to be the best one of all.

9

You could definitely call my childhood "different": filled with lots of interesting characters, the full-color palette of what you can imagine in Columbus, Georgia, circa the early 80s and with my unique challenges of larger-than-average lymph nodes, multiple surgeries, radiation, endless vomiting, something called an "ice cap" (no, not a glacier), and an early education in cancer-fighting medicines.

I told you, it was different.

However, my childhood was also filled with all the love and experiences many kids have: fishing trips, playing with G.I. Joe men and Transformers, watching cartoons, getting roughed up but never injured in neighborhood football games, having an older brother to tease and love me (and me teasing and loving him right back), going on camping trips, riding go-karts, being adored by some awesome grandparents (and one particular fantastic Granddaddy who would loom large as the most important influence in my life), running, jumping, scampering and playing with my cousins, being a ninja (okay, wanting to be a ninja), and being adored by my parents. And I'm only scratching the surface. Sick as I would become in my childhood and beyond, my early years were chock full of great times that make even better memories. My childhood was challenging and sometimes flat-out painful, but that bad stuff was balanced with love, fun, and comfort, with comfort probably the most important of all. The comfort I received from my family, friends, other patients, and medical staff would, in many ways, save my life.

I was a total goofball in my family of my older brother (by two years) Jason, my mom, and my dad. A free-spirited kid with oodles of energy and much to say about most everything, I was the one who made all of the jokes, danced like a maniac, and had fun. "Ryan... please! Do not do that at the dinner table. Don't make me tell you again," my mom would say as we ate dinner at my grandmother's house. I had a bad habit of doing everything but eating when I was a kid. I was a bundle of energy around the people I was most comfortable with.

When it came to school, on the other hand, I was an uber introvert, and it was a significant challenge for me. I remember in the first, wait, and second, oh, and third grade too, my mom walking me to the door of the classroom at Columbus Christian Academy on the first day of school, the teacher baiting me in with a piece of candy or toy. It wasn't so much that I didn't like this private Christian school my brother and I attended or that I was being bullied, at least not as early on as kindergarten. I was simply shy (beyond my grandmother's dinner table) and would often freeze up answering questions in class. Show and tell? Forget it! To get up in front of a classroom like that was flat-out terrorizing. As I think back on it now, it was probably equally painful for the kids watching me in my awkward, helpless state.

One time, I even dropped my most prized rock from my rock collection, shattering it on the hard classroom floor while trying to extricate it, terrified, for my round of show and tell.

From as far back as kindergarten, I couldn't mix with the other kids. Maybe I was just a snob, who knows? (I doubt this, though, as my family was far from rich; we were middle class at best.) But I had a hard time mingling with the other toddlers. I didn't exactly have a full grasp on the playground social scene, a hard, interpersonal, give-and-take geo-political situation at the best of times. I guess I didn't get it, or probably didn't want to get it.

I did, however, manage to track down one girl that I liked, a girl who needed me as badly as I needed her. Together we would take on the world (or our classroom, at least), traipsing across the continually shifting sands and potholes of toddler-land.

Like me, Teddy was far from a social butterfly. She was tiny, about as talkative as me (nobody ever had to tell us to be quiet), a small, fair-skinned thing with freckles. She was also a bit cross-eyed, but she was pure beauty in my eyes. I can picture her now in her tiny little dress with a delicate floral print; everything about that girl was tiny, now that I think about it. She was my perfect twin.

You couldn't call it puppy love. What we had was more a deep friendship born between two kids who recognized a personal skittishness of the world we shared. Teddy and I would get together as much as we could during our time in kindergarten. We'd only end up being friends for our first two years in school, but we were inseparable for those two years.

Our typical day was spent playing games, playing with blocks, eating snacks, and taking naps (yeah, the tough heavy-lifting life of a six-year-old). Teddy and I would always sit in the middle of the floor and people-watch as we played with our blocks. If adults were talking or if there was some commotion, we'd always look away and then right back at each other to try and figure what the other one may have been thinking. Our relationship was 99% based on these looks we gave each other; rarely did we speak. Why bother? We were painfully shy and had limited vocabularies anyway.

We spoke to each other through those looks of approval, looks of confusion, looks sometimes of a private joke shared, sneaking a smile now and then, and even an escaped giggle or two. But that's about all we did. We let the world go on around us, knowing we couldn't be part of it in the way other people were. We never once saw any imperfection in one another. We never judged what we felt or how we felt. We were comrades in arms, battling the world around us best we knew how. If only we could carry such unwavering acceptance and camaraderie into adulthood.

The other friend I made that first year of school was Andy. He was a skinny red-headed kid, quiet like Teddy and me, though Andy and Teddy never hung around together unless I was in the mix. We remained friends through third grade, after which my brother and I left our private school, then Andy and I reconnected in junior high. We'd come to play music together (drums for him, guitar for me) and get in a little trouble even. Through that modern marvel of time travel and never-ending "likes," I have managed to stay in touch with Andy on Facebook.

As my early school years passed, life got progressively harder. I took more trips to the doctor, had more surgeries and cancer treatment (all of which I will tell you about in a following chapter), plus, on top of all of that, I was a pretty small kid anyway. As an aside, in a totally unscientific, completely biased, yet newsworthy independent study conducted by Yours Truly, I found that being a small kid growing up isn't exactly an easy thing.

Fortunately, though, my dad put me in karate at an early age—my chance to practice being a ninja—and I was so glad that he did. "Never let yourself get hit first, Ryan. If someone threatens you, don't let yourself get hit. Defend yourself!" he would say. He set up a heavy bag in the garage, showed me some kicks he had learned, and bought me several karate magazines. Over time, I'd come to take Shorin-Ryu Karate briefly as a kid before getting sick again. Later, in high school and as an adult, I'd happily study Daitō-ryū Aiki-jūjutsu, Xing Yu Quan, and Taichi, until I was thirty-six and had to quit practicing them because my heart was too damaged by all the cancer treatments. I couldn't train as hard any longer; I'd get too winded.

In elementary school, though, as such a small kid and always getting challenged, I never backed down, no matter what the cost. And trust me, I most definitely paid a cost. I remember it well, my ribs remember it, and my face remembers it. Whether around the neighborhood or at school, somebody always wanted to try and "start something" with me, the small kid.

Outside of those early home karate moves, I also gained some of the best training a man (kid) could ever get. That was older-brother-kicking-your-butt-every-Saturday-morning-after-cartoons training.

My brother and I had a little ritual that went down every Saturday morning, like clockwork. We would watch our favorite cartoons, like *Super Friends*, *Smurfs*, *Flintstones*, etc., and then we would "ninja" each other. Yes, there it is again, the N-word.

At the time, my brother Jason was a higher level ninja than me. When our cartoons were over, my brother would immediately pull me off the couch as I tried to cling onto whatever I could. He would pull me to the ground and try to hold me down. Well, there was very little trying on his part; he would simply hold me down. He'd pin me down with my arms over my head, give his most evil grin, and laugh as I struggled to break away. At times he'd even do the yo-yo spit thing; this was pretty terrifying. Jason would release a steady stream of spit, and this wet string of drool would dangle in my face, and just before it touched me, my brother would *shhhulrp* it back up. Yeah, nasty stuff. Lucky for me, though, the spit never made it farther than "dangling."

"I bet you can't get me off of you... see if you can... see, you can't," he'd say in his mischievous voice. I'd lie there on the carpet in front of the TV squirming and yelling with the sound of Barney Rubble in the background. That's all I could do.

"Get off of me... Stop!" I'd scream, teetering between anger and laughter. Jason and I would fight like that until we woke my parents with our bickering and the noise of us slamming into the furniture in the living room. Yeah, we got into a little trouble, but the good thing was that Jason and I knew that if Mom and Dad were up, breakfast was right around the corner. We were about to get some "real" food, something other than Cocoa Pebbles or Raisin Bran.

Denny's or Shoney's "all you can eat!" breakfast buffet was usually how a Saturday morning ended up for us.

Now let me get this straight from the outset here. I'm not saying fighting is a good thing, but as young boys, it seems to be a rite of passage. The opportunity is always there for you to try your hand (and often your head) at it. You want to try it, and after a few pep talks and cool fighting movies, you are ready to go for it, or at least you think you are. I've always wondered how many playground fights the movie *Karate Kid* inspired.

Fighting teaches boys that whole thing about respect. Teachers, politicians, principals, and members of the politically correct, secular society, please don't lecture me here. I'm merely telling my story. I always say, walking away from a fight is best for your health and possibly your checkbook. And the basic tenet of every martial art is to not be there for the punch, as much as to avoid a fight until you have no other recourse but to fight. But nothing snaps a person into reality like being punched in the face (well, for me, anyway). And as a boy grows up, he never forgets that on a primal level, fighting could be an option when dealing with another man. You might have to fight back, and for this reason mostly, reasonable (some might say "intelligent") men never get too carried away with their words (or their fists). Most of the time.

But I was a scrawny young kid who didn't like to get pushed around. Anyway, my first punch to a human face was in first grade on the playground at Columbus Christian Academy. That's right— we Christians fight too.

There I was, finishing up a round of see-saw, nothing out of the ordinary. The next thing I knew, I saw Willie, the grade-school terrorizer. Willie never seemed to be a fan of mine. Come to think of it, Willie wasn't a fan of anybody or anything, except maybe inciting fear in other kids. The typical grammar-school bully, he was someone nobody ever liked to see on the playground, let alone run into. He was quite the character, though—a skinny black boy with quite the astonishing high-wagging afro; he might have been four foot three, but shave off that 'fro, and Willie would only have measured three foot seven, I'm sure.

On any given day, Willie would be ready to get in your face and talk some mean first-grader trash: "Man, those aren't even real Nikes," or "I bet you couldn't beat me in a wrestling match," and the simple challenge of, "You're scared." Which, of course, we all were.

Other times, Willie might make fun of your Hot Wheels or maybe make fun of your show-and-tell item. He was mean, and anything was fair game when it came to Willie and his insults: your see-saw skills, your Trapper Keeper, or even your mother. "Yo momma!" was an especially popular taunt for ol' high-haired Willie. Sure, as I've matured, I know all about how bullies are hiding behind mounds of insecurities. I know now that if you stand up to a bully, they usually back down, that their bluster is often much worse than their bite if even they end up having much of a bite at all. But at the time, I was a terrorized skinny little kid around Willie.

This one particular day, though, I wasn't havin' any of Willie's BS. As Willie approached me on the noisy little playground with that same old precarious smile, I just knew *it* was going to go down this day. And I was ready, even a little excited, to be honest.

My heart rate sped up. My thoughts raced. But I was ready to "ninja" this kid big time. The way I figured it, if I could take a beating from my brother Jason on a Saturday morning, not much worse would come from skinny Willie. I also remembered what my dad had told me on many occasions about not getting hit first; heck, not getting hit at all would be great by me! I felt like my dad was with me on that playground that day, and I was ready.

The next thing I knew, as expected, Willie was in my face, and a little too close if you ask me. There he stood, much taller than me, talking his trash. I don't even remember right now much of what he was saying, but I knew something had to give.

"You're a sissy," he said (okay, I do remember that part). He repeated this insult in several different variations. I have to give Willie credit, even these many years later. I realize he was one creative grammar school kid when it came to how differently he could riff on the same insult.

This encounter was a little different from any of the others we had had. There was no introductory insult to warm me up for the more threatening ones. Willie simply went straight to what he thought about me. He was going for the jugular from the outset. It was on, brother, big time.

I didn't say much. But I decided that my see-saw time was over. I headed over to the monkey bars. Maybe I wasn't as ready to confront Willie as I initially thought. It turns out, Willie walked over to the monkey bars as well, and with him came a few other kids, the usual round of spectators. They all wanted to watch and see how this situation would progress. This rogue gallery probably grew up to be loyal fans of reality TV, the UFC, and the documentary *Faces of Death*.

Once at the monkey bars, Willie approached me, his chest now touching mine. There was an eclipse; oh wait, it was his hair. Then he started in on me again; man, he did have a lot of energy to run his mouth. I believe it was the same ol' mess about me being a sissy... blah, blah, blah, but by now I was getting angry. I mean, the kid's chest was pressing on mine; I was under a big dark cloud from his 'fro; my schoolmates were gathering and could smell blood. I wondered what would happen after Willie was finished with all this talking. I knew it was time to act. The situation had reached its climax, and it was up to me to decide how it all would go from here. The pressure was on. I had to make a strong showing here, for me as much as for the entire playground.

All I could think about was Kung Fu Theater; *Karate Kid* hadn't come out yet. I also thought about the devastating punches I had delivered to my defenseless punching bag at home. I could tear that thing up. So, I fought off my nerves, suppressed the jitters (at least some of them), and let my right fist fly—BAM!

Willie was hit.

"I hit Willie! I hit Willie!" I shouted.

This was as big in my mind as Howard Cosell's famous, "Down goes Frazier! Down goes Frazier!" announcement.

Willie was knocked a few steps back. Was this the victory I had hoped? He looked at me in total surprise. Heck, everybody on the playground looked at me in complete amazement and didn't say a word.

Willie touched what he suddenly realized was a bleeding lip, glanced at me, and had no further comment. None. Trash talk shut down! He had nothing more to say, probably for the first time in his life. Getting hit is the last thing a bully ever thinks will happen.

That was it. The whole incident wasn't as grandiose as I had envisioned or maybe hoped it would be. I mean, in my head I saw the blood of Kung Fu Theater and heard the commentary that would go along with an ESPN knockout, like those I had seen many times at my granddaddy's house on Saturday nights. At any rate, though, there was blood, there was victory, and I soaked it up—the victory, not the blood.

After school, I was so excited to tell my mom that I had kicked some butt, I burst in the door, proudly proclaiming, "Mom, I punched Willie's face on the playground. I busted his lip. It was bloody!"

"What! Why did you punch Willie? What are you talking about?"

"Well, Mom, I thought he was going to punch me first. So I just did what Dad always told me to do."

Mom acted irritated, even a little disgusted about the whole Willie showdown, but she was also quite aware of Willie's impact on my playground life. Deep down I knew that she was probably proud, she just didn't want to encourage fighting. Moms usually have to take the moral high road; that's a rule taught in chapter 1 of the *Mom Handbook*.

Later that night when I told my dad, he thought it was a good idea to punch Willie. He wanted to hear about every single detail of the fight. Who said what? What did other people say after the fight? What did the teacher say? Did I get into any trouble?

To be honest, I felt a little sorry for Willie. Willie, if you are out there, sorry about the lip, man.

So, chalk one up for the little kid standing up for himself. Take a lesson from this or not. I'm just saying that defending myself for the first time—and yes with my fists, I admit that—was a seminal moment in my growing up.

As I mentioned, we weren't rich, but we weren't poor either. We lived in a little house in Columbus, Georgia, the same town where most of my relatives lived. Dad was the breadwinner, working as a computer programmer for Blue Cross/Blue Shield (BCBS would later be the one to publish my first book). My mom worked as a part-time secretary at Columbus Christian Academy, the same school Jason and I went to early on. She would continue to do this on and off throughout my childhood and into my teens, best she could, while driving us hours all around the state for my treatments and diagnosis. My mom was and is a rock, really. She'll be weighing in here soon.

I lived a normal existence, beyond my health troubles. We rode skateboards (a lot), shot BB guns, played army. I had many friends. My dad's sister and her husband had a house "in the country," as we called it, where my brother, mom, dad, and I would often go to play with my cousins. They had all kinds of animals and tons of space to run around. It was so great. We went there often, and we also spent time at my mom's brothers' houses with their kids and at both sets of my grandparents' homes. My mom's mom was the quintessential Southern cook; we ate great when we visited her. And my dad's father, Granddaddy Hamner, who looms large in my story and even gets his own chapter later, had a pool at his house, and we all spent lots of times there. It was like the meeting place for that side of the family.

We were all close and, while there was the usual interplay and drama between personalities, everybody got along great; there was great comfort all around. That "C" word was pretty important to me, and I needed the comfort of having my family around me.

Oh yeah, about cancer... Between the ages of three and five, I suffered from swollen lymph nodes on my neck, ear infections, pneumonia, and constant infections. A prominent doctor in my town (some might accurately replace the word "prominent" with "arrogant") insisted these symptoms were from allergies only; he got down on my mom for bringing me in so much. But when I turned five, a family friend from Puerto Rico, Dr. Rivera, said we should get to Emory Hospital in Atlanta to have me checked out. We drove the two hours to Emory, where I saw Dr. Andrews and had some tests. A few months later I had surgery on my neck and was diagnosed with Hodgkin's lymphoma.

I mention my diagnosis because clearly it was a huge part of my childhood. But even though I was pretty sick as a kid and faced some serious issues, I also had a wonderful, rich childhood filled with everything a kid could ask for: a close, loving family, many adventures, and wild characters who would come to influence me in so many great ways.

Chapter 2

I Was Squanto—But Only for a Day

In everything give thanks.

–I Thessalonians 5:1

Many of the difficult events in life are ones that we choose to experience. Maybe it's taking a certain job, deciding whether or not to have kids, choosing the best financial options for the future or what college to go to, asking somebody out on a date, or breaking up with someone. All these decisions can be stressful, but at the same time, they are choices.

What about those instances where we don't have a choice? What about those "opportunities" we can't say no to, we can't turn down, we can't change, not even a little bit? Some might call it fate, karma, or one of those all-too-real and ready "stuff happens" moments. I call it "God's plan." We all know that plenty of events come down the old bowling alley of life to knock our pins down that we can't stop or avoid.

Well, one of these opportunities is getting cancer. And yes, it *is* an opportunity. It's an opportunity to gain perspective—to learn value and appreciate the little moments, the people in your life, and to realize how temporary our lives truly are.

I was around three years old when I first experienced the symptoms associated with cancer. My mom and dad spent a significant amount of time taking me back and forth to the local doctor's office in our hometown in a never-ending nightmare of confusion for everyone involved. The aforementioned arrogant doctor couldn't diagnose me and after a time didn't even seem to care what was truly wrong with me. Even though I was constantly suffering from swollen lymph nodes in my neck, infections, and pneumonia, the attitude, vibe—call it whatever you like—that I felt from this prominent doctor, even as a little kid, was that every time my mom brought me into his office, he would think, "Oh Jeez, here we go again, not this kid again?" You tell me: if you generally don't like kids and don't have a gentle bedside manner, why would you ever become a pediatrician?

Each time, the guy would assure my parents I was suffering from cat allergies and would tell me to take Benadryl or would give me yet another prescription that would be equally ineffective. Man, I pretty much felt like crap 24/7, and nothing this doctor did helped, least of all his attitude.

As my mom remembers:

> *Ryan suffered through many infections, over and over. He'd get sick at school, his kindergarten class, at home. One time he woke up with the right side of his face swollen, as if he had fallen and hit his cheek, but I knew he hadn't. And every time we'd take him to see the doctor, the man dismissed Ryan's symptoms. He just said it was what*

happened to little boys; they get swollen glands, etc. The last comment I remember hearing from the man, who spoke loudly and angrily at me, was: "It's only one child in a million that ever has anything serious!" To which I responded: "What if Ryan is that one child in a million?"

He was one in a million to me!

Pretty much from there, I was in a panic to get Ryan's records transferred to a new local doctor in our hometown of Columbus, Georgia, so we could get a referral to Emory in Atlanta. At that time, a patient had a much more difficult time requesting records and getting them transferred to another doctor; laws have changed in this way, thankfully. During this process, Dr. Rivera (our friend and minister at one time) visited and confirmed what I already sensed, that it was critical for Ryan to see a specialist, and we should not delay getting him seen by someone qualified to make a real diagnosis.

It was another week before we could get an appointment with the new local pediatrician, who immediately made the referral to Emory. He, too, thought that Ryan should see the doctors at Emory. During this appointment, I was able to glance at the "records" transferred and saw that they consisted of only two typewritten pages. I immediately felt a lump in my throat, as I guessed that my son's medical records had been "washed" by an incompetent doctor with no care about Ryan's health.

Emory Pediatric Clinic at Egleston Children's Hospital (Children's Healthcare of Atlanta presently) is in Atlanta. As Mom says, the local doctor who got my records transferred agreed with Dr. Rivera that, yes, I needed to be in the expert care of the physicians at Egleston and Dr. Gibbs Andrews. Dr. Andrews was a pediatric surgeon who was more in tune with kids and cared much more about me than my regular doctor. He was concerned about the swelling in my neck and immediately insisted on doing a biopsy of a lymph node on the right side of my neck. Lucky for me that Dr. Andrews was so proactive, because Dr. Thad Ghim, my first pediatric oncologist, soon discovered that my problem wasn't an allergy to cats; I had Hodgkin's lymphoma.

This is a lesson to all those parents out there who instinctively know there is something wrong with their kid, even though a doctor might be telling you the opposite. Even if they are constantly trying to assure you that your child is just fine, is going through a phase, that those symptoms that seem so shocking are somehow normal (and I still don't know how my initial doctor justified all the problems I was presenting), go with your gut! Who knows your child better than you? Even if he or she is not showing obvious symptoms like I was, don't hesitate if you feel something is not right with your son or daughter. If not for my mom's face-off with my initial pediatrician (quack), who knows what might have happened?

So, the fight started. Mom, Dad, me, and even Jason would be facing cancer in one way or another. Yes, it sucked. Yes, we didn't ask for it. Yes, this is something that is horrific to consider in anyone's life, especially a five-year-old's. I don't exactly remember my parents' reaction to the diagnosis, because they kept the sadness, anxiety, and fear to themselves.

Though as I have learned from my mom:

I remember answering the first phone call from Emory Pediatric Clinic on a winter's day long ago, Christmas ornaments still scattered but slowly making their way to the attic. Ryan had just turned six that October and was sitting in my lap on our living room sofa when the phone rang. I answered to hear Dr. Ghim's voice, serious and compassionate. Laced in his deep Korean accent, he told me that my littlest one was very sick but that he could be treated. Dr. Ghim, in kindness for us both, told me that this disease was different for children and, with the protocol, chances were good for Ryan to recover. The news was heart-wrenching and life-altering. You can never forget the words that the doctor uses to tell you that your child has cancer, words that steal your breath, your joy, and make you feel as if your heart has been snatched from your soul. For a long while afterward, I stood outside the world as it went by. Every now and then, I find myself still doing this, just standing outside reality, trying to put into perspective or even to take it all in, all that Ryan has been through since such an early age. But from right then and there, hanging up the phone, holding my sick child who had no clue right then what was attacking his little body, I set it in my mind that we would

beat this. I resolved that my son would be okay. I refused
to believe anything else. I would accept no other outcome.
In fact, there was no other outcome than my son surviving.

I knew my folks were worried, then as much as now, but man, with hindsight it kills me that the people closest to me went through such hell for so long. But as my mom says, we would beat it, although it would take many years of my life to do so.

As for my brother, I don't think he understood any of it. Heck, I looked normal. I still watched cartoons with him every morning, and he could still hold me down on the floor and yo-yo spit over my face. He was just a kid himself. He knew about as much as I did about cancer, which was nothing at all.

As I began the first blush of my treatments, we took numerous trips to the doctor. Within a matter of weeks, Dr. Andrews not only had completed a biopsy to diagnose me, but he had also performed what is called a laparotomy to *stage* the disease, to find out how far my cancer had progressed. At that time, doctors believed in the protocol of removing the spleen as a precautionary procedure, so out went my spleen. As I will reiterate plenty of times in my story, the way things were done way back when I first had cancer compared to how they are done now is like cavemen using rocks for tools as opposed to using a brand-new hammer or screwdriver you just bought from Home Depot—a world of difference. But back then, this is the way things were done, and this is what I went through.

I can remember a place in the hospital called the "procedure room." Just being inside that room, which smelled of a combination of bleach and alcohol, filled me with so much anxiety of what was to come.

"You can go with your son if you want. You don't have to, but you can," the doctor told my mom. Anytime my mom had the choice, she'd be right by my side for any procedure.

On this particular day, I can remember her going with me and standing to the side of the table where I was lying down for my bone marrow biopsy. They did this by drilling into my pelvic bone. Yeah, good times. Well, I got through that, as well as several more procedures in that room, Mom by my side as much as she could be before treatment even began.

I remember the bone marrow biopsy vividly. Honestly, many parts of my life during that time are a bit blurry, all blending in my shoddy memory. But that day, I remember lying on the cold and narrow procedure table with my head turned to the side staring at all the supplies around me—stockpiles of cotton swabs, alcohol pads, bandages, medical trays, and tools—wondering which items would be used on me. I was extremely groggy, but still, I could see my reflection in the glass door of the cabinet. As the doctor and staff prepped for the procedure, my eyes scanned each movement vigorously, analyzing and attempting to determine what was going on and when I would feel the needle. When the doctor began the procedure, I saw him bearing down, trying to get the large needle to go into my hip bone. As he would bear down, I could feel the resistance, the shaking. I lay there, watching it all in the reflection of the glass door.

Dr. Thad Ghim, who would become my primary oncologist, reassured my family more times than I can count, that, "Cancer is different in children. And yes! There are things we can do to fight this." I know those words were like a life raft to us all.

So, because I was just a kid going through what no kid should ever have to go through, my new team of doctors, who truly cared, carefully decided to limit my treatments as much as they could while still being effective. To their way of thinking, if the cancer cells did not show up in my bone marrow, we'd all take this as a positive sign, and hopefully, I might get by with only radiation treatments. After a few of those treatments to my neck and a few weeks of a break before the last of those treatments, I was back to being a normal kid. "Normal" would be only for a little more than a year, though.

Mom reminds me now that at that time, all during that year I was "cured" the first time, we'd attend remission parties. It was part of the overall therapy for kids who, like me, had gone through cancer treatment and were walking around feeling OK. It was another way for the community of cancer survivors to get together and celebrate good health. These days I know cancer survivors find one another on the net; I have even done this myself. But you have to remember that way back when, we had no access to the Internet, no social media. While the cancer community was a large one (and really, ask anybody who has had cancer, I am sure they will quickly tell you that even if they have been in remission for decades, being a member of the cancer community is something they would have gladly never been part of), the only way you would meet a fellow survivor, sufferer, or their families was at a clinic, hospital, or one of these get-togethers. I am sure they gave my parents as much a feeling of camaraderie as they did for me and the group of kids I'd play with for an afternoon.

Life was good then, being in remission. I'd sleep over at my friend Andy's house. I'd go to church lock-ins, where we slept overnight at the church, made bonfires, played games, and stayed up all night, which, as a kid, is like the best thing on earth. I'd play army. I was fishing more than ever and swimming as often as I could. I think I even owned every G.I. Joe at the time. Up until "it" came back, I was feeling quite good physically and was doing pretty much what every other kid was doing, not having to endure treatments.

But when I reached nine, my life was interrupted again; "it" was back, scarier than that clown in the sewer in that Stephen King book of the same name. Although there's never a right time for cancer, this recurrence couldn't have come at a worse time for me. I had felt strong, like I had beat the thing, that I could now be a normal kid. But this recurrence killed my spirit and took the wind out of my happy sails to have to start therapy again.

As I already mentioned, although I had no clue at the time, or maybe I sensed it but was so consumed with feeling so bad I could only focus on myself, I didn't know how all this was killing my parents. Getting cancer in the first place, then the recurrence, my mom relates now with chilling recall how devastated she was. But never at any time did she (or my dad) show their fear to me. We researched everything there was to know about this disease, which was too much for any family, and as Mom says, it never got easier; it was always the worst circumstance it could be. But all the time she would assure me that I would come out of the current round of treatments just fine. She even says that on occasion I'd ask her straight out, "Mom, am I gonna die?" to which she would always reply: "No, you're not." And when I'd follow right up by asking, "Could I die?" she'd assure me: "Yes, you could, but you are going to have this therapy, and you are going to be OK." I can't even imagine what it is like to watch your child go through this!

Once again, my family and I got into the routine of treatments, surgery, hospital visits, all the back and forth of traveling from Columbus to Atlanta. I endured a combination of chemo, then radiation, and then more chemo. I missed school, missed out on ski trips with my cousins, dealt with bouts of nausea and vomiting, never knowing just how bad I might have to feel before I could recover from the latest round of treatments. I'd be wheeled into a room at Egleston's Pediatric Clinic, which was in a new building at the time, associated with the Emory University Hospital and its full medical college campus, and sit around with a bunch of other sick kids, all waiting our turns for chemo. We'd assemble puzzles, play with the toys, and do what any normal group of kids would do together. I do recall the occasional bald kid being in the room with me, a weird sight at first but something you do, over time, get used to, best that you can. One kid in particular seemed to simply fade away right before my eyes. He went from losing his hair, then becoming bald, then losing a leg to amputation. We were all quite sick. I remember my dad asking often, "Want to go for a ride?" He didn't mean in a car. He was asking if I wanted to go for a ride in a wheelchair.

Riding in a wheelchair many times meant having a break in my monotonous day that included being in and out of sleep because of medicine that made me groggy, the pain from my stitches, and the sound of a TV playing soap operas, infomercials, and endless news—nothing that a kid would be into. Actually (and don't tell anybody), I did start getting into the soap operas. I mean, why not? For so many hours during the day, I sat there with nothing else to do, and the stories were so wild and completely improbable, a nine-year-old could get hooked.

On one particular occasion, I remember that I recently had had surgery on my stomach. Man, this was tough. Walking wasn't easy. Heck, sitting up wasn't easy, and coughing was a nightmare. I would have given anything not to have had this recurrence, and even more than anything to not have had the disease spread. But Dad loaded me up with all of my tubes into a wheelchair. We went up and down the hallways saying "hi" to the staff on the floor. He took me to all the windows on the floor and pointed out objects far out in the distance. From the upper floor, we could see the trees, parking lots, little cars, and tiny people. "In a few days that will be you out there," he'd say. And yep, he was right.

I remember I wanted to be outside in the sun so bad. I wanted to be back at school. I wanted to see the singing mechanical animals and eat some pizza down at ShowBiz Pizza, which always pulled me back in!

As we strolled the hospital hallways, we'd glance into the rooms of other kids. "You should go talk to that little boy later, Ryan. You'd probably make him feel better," my dad said that day, as he always did when he got me out like this.

Dad always wanted me to understand that other kids in the hospital might have it worse. He was never the guy to say, "Aww, poor little Ryan." It was just the opposite with him. I think for this reason I never saw myself as "poor little Ryan," which was a good thing. The last thing I needed, on top of everything else I was going through, a year shy of ten years old, was to start with the self-pity.

Staying in the hospital for any length of time was always a challenge. I think the key for my mom and dad was always to give me something to look forward to. Usually, it was, "Bamba and Granddaddy are coming to see you today!" or "Want us to go get you a goodie bag from the gift shop?" And even one time there was actually, "Hey! I got you some new underwear!" Anything could be made into something exciting. My mom eventually added ordering breakfast, lunch, and dinner into the list of exciting pastimes.

Other than getting a new G.I. Joe—I was amassing quite the collection—the most amazing thing to look forward to was the aforementioned ShowBiz Pizza.

ShowBiz had video games, skeeball, and a dancing bear. OK, about that bear. I don't really know how to describe it, but the "house band" at ShowBiz was a bunch of mechanical animals that sang songs and danced as you sat at your table and ate pizza and sang along. Interesting concept, huh? I have since learned that ShowBiz Pizzas existed all across the country. They are part of that great American tradition of pizza, video games, and slightly creepy animal animatronics called "family entertainment centers" that hit this country in the late 70s and early 80s. ShowBiz was the direct result of a corporate separation between Robert L. Brock and Pizza Time Theater (Pizza Time owned the Chuck E. Cheese franchise; "Chucky," another great musical animal—a mouse—you may have heard of).

Imagine the men and women pitching their dancing bear and pizza dream to the big money backers the first time. Now that's a corporate meeting I would have loved to have been in on.

I can clearly remember my mom saying, "When we are done here (at the doctor), we're going to ShowBiz. Just be patient." I don't remember patience as always being easy for me, and it still isn't. However, I do remember always mustering up whatever patience I could for the promise of seeing that bunch of singing, dancing mechanical animals while eating some moderately tasty pizza. The place was heaven for me and would make each trip to the hospital, each new needle prick, almost worth it. Almost.

After the chemo came more radiation. After beginning the treatments at Emory in Atlanta, the treatments were done locally, back in my hometown. I remember being so confused as to why the medical staff drew dark red lines on my neck with a smelly magic marker. These lines were used to line up the radiation machine for proper "zapping." Still attending school when I could, I do recall looking at myself in the mirror and noticing those magic marker lines while I went to class or walked down the hallway. But the teachers in school were sympathetic about what I was going through and helped me make up the work I was missing. As for my fellow students, well, back then nobody knew all that much about cancer, especially grammar school kids, so nobody confronted me about how I looked or why I was absent so much. I wouldn't have known what to say to them, anyway.

Other than Mom and Dad, I also had a champion in Miss Sydney. I met her briefly the first time I presented with cancer, at six years old; she was still working at the hospital (thank God!) when I came back at nine. The predictable schedule of hospital life would be broken up by the unpredictable Miss Sydney.

A lady in her fifties, Miss Sydney was one of sweetest women I can remember during my hospital stays. She'd sometimes dress up as a clown but always acted like a clown unless you needed her to help you through a hard day. Miss Sydney worked at both the clinic, where kids received their chemo, and at the hospital. She was a blast. She'd push around "Miss Sydney's Cart," filled with all sorts of goodies for us kids. Anytime you saw her, she'd give you a tight hug—whether you wanted it or not (although you always secretly wanted it)—then she'd offer you a surprise of some sort from her cart.

There are angels; really, that's all you can call people like Miss Sydney. They radiate light, love, and hope in a situation where you can easily lose all hope. For kids fighting cancer, for parents and caregivers dying a bit more each day that they watch their child endure surgery and chemo, a person like Miss Sydney, selflessly administering to children, knowing exactly what a kid needed even before the kid knew what he or she needed, was a lifesaver.

As I said, my cancer treatment involved many road trips. Usually it was my mom driving me back and forth two or three times a week to Egleston's Pediatric Clinic in Atlanta, Georgia, for doctor's appointments and regular chemotherapy treatments. Dad was at home most of the time working (treatment ain't cheap!), taking care of Jason, and holding down the fort. If I had a surgery or anything serious, he was always there, though. That's how I learned what was and wasn't serious. If Dad showed up, I knew something out of the ordinary was about to take place or had just taken place. If my dad wasn't there, I figured everything was going as expected, nothing to worry about, cancer business as usual.

As time went by, road trips evolved into, well, not just any ol' road trips. We had rituals like our McDonald's Egg McMuffin stop in the morning as we headed out. For some reason, we couldn't eat or stop anywhere else. Then we had the McDonald's-by-Shannon-Mall pee stop. Seriously, any other restroom would have worked perfectly fine, but for whatever reason, we always had to stop at the

McDonald's by Shannon Mall. These trips and their stops happened like clockwork. Every week, same days, same times (same bat time, same bat channel) and the same McDonald's. And no, we were not, and are not sponsored by McDonald's. I think it's the other way around, actually.

As we would get closer to Atlanta, my nerves would start going crazy. I knew what was coming up shortly. I remember that I played all kinds of weird games in my head to keep the anxiety at bay. Sometimes I'd think, "The next time I see Jason and Dad, this will be over. I will have had the treatment and be finished getting sick," or "The next time I ride my skateboard, I will have finished chemo." But no matter how I talked myself into or through the treatments, preparing myself for the violent sickness that always followed the treatment was a nightmare.

Another positive step in modern cancer treatment that wasn't even a blip on the horizon way back then is the whole host of new drugs patients can take now that significantly lessen the nausea associated with chemo treatment. Such was not the case when I was nine. I remember my mom and I would often sit outside the clinic at a picnic table while waiting for my name to be called for treatment. Sitting in the sun, I'd often be holding back the tears, dreading what was to come. I always hoped that somehow each treatment might be different than the last. That maybe this time I wouldn't get sick.

On one of these times, I found a stick with its bark peeling off. It kind of looked like a flower that needed a little more work to look like a real flower. I took out the pocket knife that I always carried with me and carved the bark down off the stick. Now it looked like a flower with petals, or at least it looked like a flower to me. Then I had an idea. I saw a tree nearby that had all sorts of crooks and crevices in it. Out of boredom, I guess, I took the stick/flower and put the end of the stick into one of the crevices.

"Mom, by the time this tree grows up around this flower stem, I'll be done with all of my treatments," I said.

This became our new marker, our gauge for how much time I had left for treatment. So every time I went for treatment, we'd check the stick/flower.

"Mom, doesn't it look like the tree is growing around my flower?" I'd say.

Thinking back, it was kind of ridiculous, I guess, but for some reason, it gave me something to look forward to. And we checked on the stick/flower long after my treatments were finished. It did eventually grow into the tree. As anybody who has ever gone through cancer or as a caregiver who has been witness to the struggle of the disease, you know how sometimes the most mundane facets of life can give you strength.

When my name was finally called for treatment, we would get up and slowly head back to the chemo room. When we reached the chemo room, usually a tall nurse by the name of CJ would meet us at the door. He was a super nice guy, and like Miss Sydney always did, he'd hug you and try to cheer you up. God knew, though, there wasn't any cheering me up at that stage of the game.

"This will be one more treatment down, Ryan. You are getting there. Next thing you know, it will all be over. Are you ready?" he would ask.

I had mixed feelings about this whole thing. Here CJ was being as nice as he possibly could. He was trying to give me a pep talk and be my friend, but at times I felt like I was being coerced into a three-hour stay in hell. I fell for the same trick every single time. Smile. Hug. Vomit. Repeat.

As I entered the chemo room, I'd see all the other kids going through chemo too. Some seemed to be doing better than others. It was just never anything that I got used to. I couldn't help but find myself staring at the other kids, wondering about their stories and how they felt at that moment. Were they scared? How did treatment make them feel?

CJ would lead me to a chair where he would start my IV and strap my wrist to an arm board. Then he would start that nasty stuff: CHEMO. It came in all different size syringes and colors. Some of the ones with the brightest, coolest colors were the ones that made you the sickest.

Treatments seemed to take forever, and the side effects were awful; no secret there. I'd get anxious, depressed, nauseous, and of course impatient. This would go on all afternoon. This was when my Walkman and some tapes my brother and I recorded would come in handy (we'll get to our recording session story in a bit). I'd listen to my favorite songs for a while, and that would help for some of the time, but not for the whole time, unfortunately. After awhile, the calming ability of the music wore off. The ability to look ahead and be excited about a G.I. Joe would wear off. Miss Sydney dropping by with toys would have absolutely zero effect on me. I would become indescribably sad, anxious, and depressed.

This is when my mom would spend endless time coaching me through the rest of the treatment. It's that last bit of a struggle in any situation where you need a mental push from someone other than yourself. I was just a nine-year-old kid who was scared, sick, and tired, but I knew this all had to be done. So I did it. The whole process from leaving the house in the morning, to stopping at the gas station, to stopping at McDonald's, and of course arriving at the clinic were just incremental steps of dread with a few glimpses of joy. And it all came to its culmination in these last few moments of treatment with my mom sitting with me holding my hand.

After finishing the day's treatment, Miss Sydney and my mom would wheel me out to the car in a wheelchair. I would be delirious from all the chemo and would tell every single person I passed on the way out either "Hi!" or "Bye!" It's kind of funny when I think on it now, this nine-year-old all goofy from chemo treatment being so jovial.

After I was buckled into the passenger's seat, I'd almost always promptly vomit. Then we'd hurry straight over to the Ronald Mc-Donald house. Yeah, there's that McDonald's again.

So much driving back and forth from home to my treatments took its toll. Luckily, we had the Ronald McDonald House. There are many of these houses around the country, staffed by volunteers, which are places for families to stay where they can bed down, be safe and comfortable, stay close to a treatment center or clinic, and save on the wear and tear of driving so many miles from their home to wherever their child is being treated. The house in Atlanta was a cozy little place tucked away in a small patch of woods right around the corner from the clinic. It had everything that any other cozy house would have, including a living room, kitchen, and of course my favorite, the playroom, which was usually entirely freed up because most of the kids staying there were not up for playing or couldn't be around others because of a temporarily suppressed immune system.

I would lie in bed from the afternoon through the night, and my whole body would shake as I heaved continuously; luckily lunch usually was something light, like cheese and crackers. I couldn't stand. I couldn't walk. I couldn't eat, and I could barely drink. I remember just lying there falling in and out of sleep, my mom wiping my mouth with a warm rag, the phone ringing with family checking in on me, and a surreal feeling of dread that never seemed to completely go away. Maybe it was the drugs, who knows. The weird thing is, it also felt normal to me. The people who stayed in the house all had their own story, but we all had the same fight, getting through cancer. After our night at the Ronald McDonald House, the next morning my mom and I would pack up and head out. This, of course, was my favorite part, because the worst was over, temporarily anyway, and we were on the way home.

Going back, we'd often make my favorite stop of all: a pick-out-a-G.I.-Joe stop at Toys R Us. From this one stop, I picked up new friends with names like Cobra, Snake Eyes, Storm Shadow, Grunt, etc. My Joe collection told the story of how many trips I had made to Atlanta.

The trips to treatment, the ups and downs of how I felt—some days pretty good actually, other days puking and tired—made me want to get back to some sort of normal life for an ordinary nine-year-old kid. And, it all made me focus on the stuff far and away from the hospital. Even things like a third-grade school play became a more significant experience in my life.

Our play that year for history class was going to be held outdoors. An off-Broadway (so "off" the cast was made up of third-graders and the play was happening in a tiny private school in Columbus, Georgia) Thanksgiving celebration, with Indians and pilgrims, where I was set to play "Squanto," an Indian. I had the costume already, even the face paint, as Squanto was a favorite character of mine.

There was one problem with this little play, however. It was to be on a day that I would be coming back from Atlanta, weak from chemotherapy.

"Mom, can we just skip this time? One time won't hurt. I want to be Squanto," I tried to reason.

"Sorry, honey, we have to go, but maybe if we are back in time and you feel like it, you can still be Squanto for the play," she replied.

The day of the play came. I slowly rolled out of my bed at the Ronald McDonald House following the previous day's treatment. I was ready to rock the role of Squanto. The day before, my treatment had included a strong dose of chemo (when were they not strong?) followed by a very rough evening, a "heavening" if you will (that's "heave" + "evening").

As we got moving, I was definitely feeling the effects of the fluids they had pumped through my IV the day before, those chemicals that were often funny colors and burned my veins. It was often referred to as "medicine," but man, this medicine always seemed to make me feel sick. Heck, the stuff made people's hair fall out! I can remember one time when my IV blew out and the chemo leaked out into my arm. It was so painful and burned for days. My arm became red and discolored. It was so bad, I had to have it wrapped. Even to this day, I can still see faint scars from that chemo mishap.

At any rate, I was really excited that there was a chance I might make it back home in time to be Squanto in the school play.

"Ryan, don't push yourself if you don't feel well. You'll only make yourself sicker," Mom said this time, as she had so many others. This was her standard line as she would come to try and temper my little-kid enthusiasm or impatience, me always wanting to do stuff above and beyond the treatments, even when I was not physically capable.

This day she was battling my childhood thespian aspirations. Heck, I was Squanto. I had to be Squanto. I was going to be Squanto!

As we set out on the road coming back from my treatment, I fell in and out of sleep. I was so worn out, exhausted, and dehydrated. I woke up when Mom pulled into a gas station, almost forcing me out of the car for a restroom break, as she usually did, even if we didn't need gas. But man, it was all I could do to keep my eyes open each time I got out of the car. I was so beat that day. Still, Squanto awaited.

"Mom, what time is it? Are we gonna make it?" I asked, managing to pop my chin from my chest when we were still a good hour away from home.

We had to make it back home by lunch; the play began at noon. That would be my time to shine as one cool little Indian, if only we could make it.

When the clock hit eleven thirty, we were still a few miles out, but I was determined to be that Indian Squanto.

"Hurry, Mom! They are going to start without me! I'm Squanto. My part is pretty important," I said, envisioning my mother as Burt Reynolds speeding down the road in *Smokey and the Bandit*.

Luckily, we had planned ahead, or my mom/Burt had. She had packed my costume and even my face paint in the car. No fancy dressing room for me.

As we rolled into town, the dashboard clock hit noon on... the... dot. I couldn't sit still. I was going to be an Indian. Finally! Me! Squanto!

When we pulled into the schoolyard, my classmates and teacher saw me. They were on a nearby playground getting ready for the outdoor play. We all knew it was go time, I just needed a few moments to "Indianize" myself. I jumped (best I could) out of our car, and my teacher, Mrs. Hodges, smiled and said: "Ryan, great! You made it! How are you feeling?" She was always great with the kids, a real sweet lady, in her midtwenties at the time, I guess, single and recently out of college. She seemed to love us like her own kids and did everything she could to show it. You have to love those enthusiastic young teachers who see so much promise in their classroom, who show such caring. Even though I wasn't in school as much as I had wanted to be or could be, ladies like Mrs. Hodges enriched my life, as would the play on this day.

As the play started, I began to get a little nervous. Strike that, I was a lot nervous, and that's a lot with a capital, A LOT. I think those nerves counteracted the exhaustion I was feeling, though, which was a good thing. I remember sitting behind the stage wall in the sun waiting for my part. I felt so good. I had made it to the play. I was Squanto.

"Andy, are you ready?" I whispered to my longtime friend.

"I think so. Do you remember all of your lines?" he asked, squinting as the sun shined in his eyes.

I had immediately stepped from one surreal, dismal world into another entirely different place. It was kind of like living between two different dimensions, not to sound all crazy or anything. But just twenty-four hours earlier I had been in a state of depression, physical exhaustion, nausea, vomiting, and tears. But right then, in the bright sunshine of a brand-new day, I was sloughing off all the bad stuff (or putting those feelings somewhere), jumping back into the role of the normal life of a nine-year-old kid. Not that being an Indian was normal, or my mom heavy-footing it down the streets of Georgia was normal, but I was a kid at school, acting in a school play outside, hanging out among my classmates and teacher, just being who I should be at that age. I was pretty dadgum happy at the moment, I can tell you that.

Because of all my treatments as a kid, I missed a lot of time at school. This was usually because my immune system wasn't strong enough to be around other kids at school or because I was sick. Okay, maybe I faked it some days, too. Give me a break. Because of these health issues, I had a teacher, Miss Bowles, who came to my home pretty often for homeschooling.

"Ryan, look at you. You're lookin' so good," she'd say, stepping through the front door of my house with a big smile on her face. Whether it was true or not (probably not), these were words I needed to hear. This was Miss Bowles. She made you feel normal when everything around you was anything but normal.

Miss Bowles was probably in her midforties, always so well dressed, super sweet, and outgoing. I friggin' loved her. I remember she was a tall black lady, but considering I was approximately four foot nothing, "tall" here is a matter of perspective. She always had on lots of perfume and, don't get me wrong, it smelled nice, but boy, did that lady wear perfume.

We'd sit at the dining room table and work on all the normal subjects: English, math, science, and history. We even worked on me, or more precisely Miss Bowles always worked hard to lift my spirits. She hugged me on the way in and on the way out. She was always in a good mood and always made our lessons (yeah, schoolwork at home, how fun is that?) as fun as she possibly could. I never thought I'd look forward to doing homework, but with Miss Bowles I did.

My life at that point was pretty crazy. All the traveling, treatments, trials, and tribulations of being a kid with cancer. Let me tell you, at times I was too scared to think straight or too exhausted to move, or both. And I know Mom and Dad, even my brother, were going through hell not knowing from one day to the next what my health was going to be like, how I would respond to a treatment, and when I may or may not be able to go home. But the people other than my family who cared for me in the most trying moments in my life, people like my teachers and classmates, the wonderful staff at the hospitals and the Ronald McDonald house, pretty much everybody who would see me and give me a smile or make me laugh or act alongside me during a school play, they made my life bearable. I wish I could thank every one of them personally. I know I made it through because of you.

Chapter 3

Music Made Me before I Made Music

Opportunity often comes disguised in the form of misfortune,
or temporary defeat.
–Napoleon Hill

Music, I've loved it ever since I can remember, and I've always been surrounded by it. As a baby, I remember my mom picking me up from my nap, holding me in her arms, and dancing with me around the living room as the stereo played loudly. I know, sounds mushy, right? But it is true. It was a great feeling. I can remember the sun shining through the curtains covering the backyard window, while the sounds filled my ears and I was held so close. We danced to whatever tune my mom had on the record player: the Beatles, Honeytree, Elton John, old country music like Kenny Rogers, you name it. Life was good, really good.

I can distantly remember my dad playing guitar, harmonica, piano, and banjo at around the time I was six or so, around the same time cancer came singing its nasty tune the first time in my life. I loved the sound of any instrument I heard. I can remember opening up my dad's guitar case and looking at the guitar, marveling over all its pieces—the frets, the strings. I remember the smell of the wood and, most importantly, I remember wanting so badly to be able to make something happen with that guitar. But at that time, I couldn't seem to figure out how to play it. How was my dad doing all of that finger-pickin' on the guitar? How could he hear songs and play them without reading music? How was he weaving this magic that made me feel so good? Man, he made it look easy.

"Do you recognize that? It's from a movie. Do you know which one?" my dad would ask as he played. He especially liked to play movie themes and songs from commercials.

"Wait, play it again, but do it slower," I'd say, watching and listening much closer the second time around.

I was amazed by everything that my dad played and wanted in on how he was able to make this magic with his fingers. For the time being, however, I would have to admire everything and take it in. So I did.

My brother Jason was also pretty crazy about music, but not exactly into playing it, which was cool; we each had our own interests, as siblings should. Jason would go on to be more interested in being an athlete. He'd forget playing music for collecting baseball cards and playing sports in general. He'd eventually get into weightlifting and end up wrestling in high school, so those pursuits took up much of his time. But he always loved hearing good songs. Athletes need good music too, right?

On Sunday nights, right after dinner, my brother and I would sit by the radio with a blank tape listening to Casey Kasem's "American Top 40." We had our tape inserted into the "jam box" ready to go. We'd wait for our favorite songs, and wait, and wait, and when one of our favorites came on, as Casey began to introduce the tune, we'd shout, "Go!" We wanted to make sure we pressed the jam box record button as soon as possible to record as much of the song as we could. We worked this recording thing like a job. It was crucial to time the song with our friend Casey and get as much of it down to tape as possible. I know with downloads, searching YouTube with an iPhone, streaming, and all of our modern instant musical gratification gizmos, acquiring music by trying to capture your favorite nugget with a ready blank tape and scrambling to push "record" seems so ancient. I guess you'd call it quaint (and I realize that many people under a certain age won't even know what I am speaking about here). But back in the day, this is what most young kids were doing before they were old enough to go out and buy a single or an album. Even older kids were taping off the radio to save a few bucks on having to buy music.

However, the recording wasn't the end of the job. There were two of us and one tape. So the next step was dubbing a copy, or making two tapes with our dad's dual cassette deck that could hold two tapes and record from one to the other. This was hi-tech at the time and highly sought-after technology. Machines like a double deck player/recorder were not cheap, and if a kid was lucky enough to have one in the house or maybe an older sibling had acquired one, you'd be dubbing to your heart's content. This recording of songs from the radio and dubbing became a regular hobby of Jason and mine and a great way for us to get our favorite tunes.

Sorry to all those eighties bands, I'm sure we owe you a few dollars in royalties.

This weekly recording ritual helped to further develop my love of music. With my tapes, I could now listen to my favorite songs over and over.

Reinforcement of melody, beat, lyric, singing, and playing met and mashed into my heart and head, and lucky for me that it did; music would come to see me through so much.

During many chemo sessions at the ages of nine and eleven, which could be hours long and made worse by those drugs that would depress me, music would lift me up. I'd have my dubbed tape playing on my Walkman nonstop. Sitting there in the dimly lit chemo clinic, the corridors saturated with the smells of medical products, smells that, to this day, I will never forget and luckily don't smell on a regular basis, I was wrapped in warm blankets, but never warm enough. I'd try to take my mind away, but at the back of my thoughts was my dread of what was coming, having been through the ritual of treatment too many times by then. Those tunes playing in my ears took me away, distracted me, and made me feel alive when I was shaking in my Pro Wings (Payless brand shoes) or holding back my tears. This attachment to music, its absolute salvation of me, how it made me *feel* the possibility of a life beyond that treatment clinic was the beginning of something that would change my life forever. Music helped to make me, as I would one day make music. It could counteract any harmful drug that had to be put into my system and would embolden me in a way nothing else could.

Around the age of fourteen, I was three years into remission from my third bout of cancer. Life was not too bad. I was finally going to school without having to use any homeschooling due to illness. I had friends; life was as normal as it could be, and I started digging into the guitar.

I became obsessed with the instrument. I got myself a chord book, tore out a page of guitar scales I found in an old *Guitar Magazine*, and every single day, I was either playing or was up the street at my friend Jamie's house watching him shred his electric guitar.

"Wait. Do it again. Slower so I can see what you are doing," I'd say. So, Jamie would then shred in slow motion.

As I have mentioned, Dad had always been "a picker, a grinner, a lover, and a . . ." Never mind. If you don't know the song, it won't much matter to you. But beyond Dad's abilities, Jamie played something I'd never seen played in person, something I only ever heard on the radio. Jamie played electric guitar, wailing through all of the popular solos of the most well-known artists. He played the music of Slash, Jimmy Page, and Stevie Ray Vaughan, masters of their craft, men who could make a guitar scream, cry, and whine. I was blown away by watching this kind of playing right in front of my face.

Inspired by what Jamie showed me, I was ready to push myself even more.

I'd come home from school, go straight to my room, and break out the nylon-string guitar that my dad had loaned me, and get to work. And on the weekends, if you wanted to find me, I'd be in my room practicing chords and scales: G, C, D, and so on. OK, so I wasn't a "Master of the Telecaster," I wasn't even playing electric guitar, but I was on my way.

"Don't you want to get up and get outside for a little bit? You've been here all day." I can't tell you how many times my mom asked me this. Ordinarily, I'd be finding things to do outside in the back-yard, riding my bike down the street or practicing moves on my skateboard, but I had found that I could do something that spoke to my soul, and I could do it on an instrument called a guitar.

Learning guitar was a bit frustrating at first, but pretty soon, it was all coming together. I knew all of my chords, I knew enough scales to rock out a little bit, and I could even play along with songs.

"Dad, listen, know what that is?"

Now it was me doing what my dad had done with songs that he had played for me.

"No, son, I don't recognize it. Keep practicing," he'd often say, smiling over how hard I was trying and how much he could obvi-ously see me loving my guitar.

Now, I'm not saying anything I was playing at that time was pretty or even technically correct, but I was playing. I'd lock myself in my room, crank up my CD player, and go to town. I played along with Guns n' Roses, SRV, the Allman Brothers, and Lynyrd Skynyrd, and interestingly enough, these great artists played right along with me. I loved it! I mean, nothing will make you sound better than playing along with a CD or a record. Even if you make mistakes, the band covers for you. I had discovered something I would never put down.

Like I mentioned earlier, I was pretty introverted in many ways. It was as much cancer waylaying me during some crucial stages of my childhood as the fact that I guess I was destined to be more of the contemplating, quieter type. Over the years I had learned how to come out of my shell somewhat, and God knows cancer certainly affected my perspective on life, good and bad. But as a kid, if you had told me that one day I'd be singing in front of people and playing my guitar, I would have laughed in your face. As it turned out, though, a year or so after learning to play guitar, I figured out that I would probably need to learn to sing and write songs since I would probably never be a Jimi Hendrix, SRV, or Slash. This was a disappointing discovery, actually, but being brutally honest with myself, I realized I would never be a rock god when it came to playing the guitar.

Speaking of rock gods, I remember watching the performance of one guitarist in particular that made my eyes grow wide, my face freeze, and at times made me even think my TV would melt: Eric Johnson's guitar playing on *Austin City Limits*. It was un-frickin' real. But as a fourteen-year-old kid just getting started with guitar, I had no idea what I was watching. Now, I know I've never played like Eric Johnson and will never be able to play like him, but this guy kept me motivated to keep practicing scales on the purple Ibanez electric guitar I eventually bought. I got a great deal on it along with a Peavey amp I purchased at the same time.

I also began singing. Well, we'll just call it "singing" for now. I believe the first song I learned to sing was "Wish You Were Here" by Pink Floyd. I then moved on to "Knocking on Heaven's Door," "Patience," and "Brown Eyed Girl"—all classics in their own way and tunes I could strum my acoustic gutar to, sing along with, and make sense of, or more importantly, songs that other people could make sense of, knew rather quickly, even at the beginning of my career when I wasn't singing them so well. I'd hang out with my friends from school on the weekends and play guitar and sing for them. I always carried my guitar with me, always ready to perform. Many times we'd all go to the lake, make a fire to sit around, and I would play. The only light around was from the moon, stars, and the fire. We'd sit there, maybe gossip a little, soaking up the night and camaraderie. This is how my weekend nights went in Georgia, and they were glorious.

Other times we'd hang out at someone's house outside in the backyard, or we'd hang out in an empty school parking lot. I freely admit, I'm sure I sounded pretty awful back then, but it all worked at the time. Nobody was judging me, and I wasn't out to prove anything to anyone, except to myself. In the amateur teenage rock and roll world, singers are usually given a lot more breaks than guys and girls trying to wail on guitar. Guitar players are like the fastest gun in town, everybody always trying to face off against them or criticize. I was getting better quietly, day by day, and most of my friends were supportive (why not, free entertainment, right?) and all the good feelings I was getting back (and sensing the improvements I was making) motivated me to keep on keeping on.

At the age of sixteen, I wrote my first song. It was called "Rain Sometimes Falls from Blue Skies," and I wrote it with my fishing buddy, Jared.

Jared and I spent many summers fishing, frog "giggin'," and playing guitar. Jared and his brother Jason always pushed me to sing, and without their encouragement, I'd probably never have sung on my own. I was way too shy. The brothers were my first real critics, outside of my own family, and were encouraging; I trusted their judgment implicitly.

Jared and I sweated out the lyrics to our opus, mainly working over the chorus. We wanted it to be absolutely perfect.

"Look, I'm telling you, that doesn't even make sense," I'd say about a particular line we were trying to write.

"Ryan, it rhymes and fits perfectly into the chorus," the Lennon to my McCartney would offer.

We struggled a bit, but we did finish. When we were done writing the song, Jared and I rounded up his family, brother, girlfriends, and sang it for the assembled. I remember everyone coming into the living room where Jared and I were sitting on the ledge of the fireplace, both smirking at each other a bit, and me rubbing my palms on my jeans nervously as we gave each other that look of, "You ready?"

It was an indescribable feeling singing and playing the first song I co-wrote. That was an especially good time and something that as much marked my friendship with Jared as has helped me up the ladder to real musical respectability. Jared and I were very proud of "Blue Skies" when we finished it, but we never got around to recording it, and the song was criticized a bit by a high school friend who said: "When does rain ever even fall from blue skies?" Yeah, everybody's a critic. But you know, ever since then I've looked for a blue sky that lets out a few rain drops here and there. I swear I've seen it happen.

In 1994, things would change for me big time. One of the key figures in my life, my Granddaddy Hamner, would succumb to emphysema. (I devote a whole chapter to this wonderful man a bit later in my story.) At seventeen years old, just after my granddaddy died, I sat down with tears in my eyes and wrote my first "real" song about the man who used to pick me up from school in his '64 Corvette when I was sick. The man who used to see me in the hospital with a smile on his face no matter what the situation. The man who could hold me captive with his incredible army stories. The list of what my Granddaddy Hamner gave me in my life spiritually, emotionally, and through memories is immeasurable, and I wanted to write a song for him.

Throughout a night, a long, late, sad night, I wrote "So Soon." It would come to be released on my first commercial record in 2007 by Mighty Loud Records, and I was quite proud of this song. Every time I hear it, I think of my Granddaddy Hamner and even feel a bit of the sting from that awful day in 1994 when I found out he had passed away.

The pre-chorus from the song says it all, "As the seasons will change, time will rearrange, the things you wanted to remain," and that's precisely what happened. This is what seems to happen in life always, I feel.

Out of high school, I pursued my musical ambitions full time. The more I played, sang, and wrote, solo and with bands, the better I became. It was the old "practice makes perfect" rule. In fact, my first real professional experience was jumping out of the frying pan and into the fire, playing and singing with a band in front of a packed house at a local bar.

Petrified?

Sure.

Hooked for life?

You bet!

I really hit the bars then, playing standards and covers. I even landed a steady gig at Picasso Pizza in Columbus, a great gig where lots of people would come in and have a slice before heading out for the night to the bars in town. I played outside the place; it was perfect for me. Really, a performing musician can only learn his chops by performing, so the more I performed, the better I became. It felt good. I liked the attention, I liked having my songs heard, and I liked making money. It was great being a professional musician.

Back in 2007, when MySpace was still kind of rockin' in popularity, I put up a couple of songs and was emailed by somebody who knew country music artist Sammy Kershaw. Sammy has released sixteen albums, has three RIAA platinum certifications and two gold certifications to his name, and has had more than twenty-five singles enter the Top 40 on Billboard's Hot Country Songs chart.

Mr. Kershaw was a big deal, not someone I thought I'd ever get close to in my meager career at that point (and my career was a career with a little 'c'). At first, I figured this person contacting me was just somebody pulling my leg, but Sammy's friend persisted and finally did convince me that Sammy liked my song "Country Club Superstar" and wanted to possibly record it.

Sammy emailed me his number. We discussed the song in detail, one he described as "mailbox money." In other words, I sit back and collect on his recording. Unfortunately, though, nothing ever came of this opportunity even after a few rewrites for Sammy.

From there I connected with Jesse Dupree, the founder, songwriter, and singer for the rock band Jackyl. Jesse had founded a record label called Mighty Loud Records, and through some fits and starts and Jesse's always warm encouragement, he invited me to be on his label.

Now lots of people started to get involved. Jesse lined up co-writers and performance opportunities, and I put out my EP on his label in 2007 and then a full album after that. I recorded the majority of the album in Atlanta at Cock of the Walk Studios. I began to open for acts in Atlanta and was contacted by an agent in Mobile, Alabama, who had me come out there to play in several venues. I was doing well, had a solid support team around me, and my view was that I was making significant progress

I had some phenomenal players recording in the studio with me. Charlie Starr from Blackberry Smoke played guitar on my songs "The View," "How You Say," and "What About Us." And keyboard player Joey Huffman, drummer Mike Froedge, and bassist Joshua Sattler put down some grooves as well. These guys were solid in the studio, super talented, and easy to work with. Then there was the man who put it all together—a true artist—none other than Jeff Tomei. Jeff had worked with Smashing Pumpkins, Matchbox Twenty, and Edwin McCain, among others. The guy was a machine who ran on Twizzlers and an occasional bottled water. He was the real deal and pushed me in the studio.

"Nope, you can do better. Let's sing it one more time," Jeff would say. I learned so much recording my record. It made me musically better in every way.

In addition to my music, in fact, before all my playing professionally and record business dealings, I had written a book back in 1999, put out by Blue Cross. It was a children's book called *You'll Be All Right, Buddy!*, an educational storybook for children with cancer. My songs, tending to the inspirational, simply furthered what I had learned and written about in that book. More than slightly sick of playing "Margaritaville" at bar gigs (sorry Jimmy B.), and Mighty Loud only committing to my one record, I presented an idea to a money person/friend about touring hospitals spreading my message through song and sharing my story.

This gig was called the "Hear the Heart" tour, and I managed to get a friend on board to sponsor me, pay for a publicist, and set me up on a rewarding tour where most of the time I was setting up my own gear. I loved it, every bit of it. I made little if any money from it, but it was all me, grassroots playing live for people who

understood and were inspired by what I had to say, as much me
being inspired by them right back. I played all the major hospitals
and cancer centers in the south and southeast: Emory University,
the University of Texas MD Anderson Cancer Center, Mary Bird
Perkins Cancer Center, the University of Alabama at Birmingham,
many "Hope Lodges" (American Cancer Society's own version of
Ronald McDonald House), and so many more places. On quite a few
occasions I'd come into some clinic or get up on a stage the hospital
had set up for me and look out onto a sea of people who wanted
to hear me sing and speak for the next hour about as much as they
wanted another round of chemo. But always I'd turn them around,
people of all ages, ethnicities, and in all stages of cancer coming up
to me after my performance to tell me how much my being there
had meant to them. That was worth more than any money I could
ever have made for that tour.

"You're our singer tonight?" an older, fragile-looking lady asked
me in Atlanta, Georgia, one night where I was playing an event.

I had just played my song "Survivors Survive." We were both
standing at the dessert table getting a slice of cake after dinner. She
must have been in her eighties but was very sharp.

"Yes ma'am, I am," I replied.

"Did you know I'm a survivor too?" she asked while staring at
me proudly with a smile. "I was supposedly terminal but have been
cancer-free for ten years now."

This was just one more story of where what would have been
expected didn't match the reality. For example, twelve years ear-

lier, during my bone marrow transplant, I met a guy named Chris while living in the Winn Dixie Hope Lodge in Atlanta, Georgia. He was in his twenties, muscular, a Navy SEAL, in fact. He was a flat-out tough guy, no doubt about it. We arrived at the American Cancer Society Winn-Dixie Hope Lodge at the same time and met right after checking in. His mom and my mom met and talked a bit, and Chris and I did our own thing. We spoke over standard stuff and then, of course, got into a discussion about our cancer. Again, I don't remember many specifics (although I do remember Chris well), but I believe that Chris also had Hodgkin's lymphoma, and I believe it was his first time up to bat with it.

"Do you actually have a donor?… Or are you your own donor?… I forget what it's called," he said. "Yeah, I'm going to have my own new bone marrow put right back into me."

Like I mentioned, Chris was fit, lean, and in very good shape. Navy SEALs are serious about their physical conditioning, and this guy looked the part for sure! A guy like this could just simply outrun cancer and be done with it, I thought. Give it a beating like an alpha male should. But, following his transplant, Chris would have complications and would not make it. Believe me, I have wondered plenty of times why a guy like Chris didn't live and I did. I always assumed if anyone would make it through cancer, of any type, he would.

For many things in my life, my expectations of how things would turn out veered drastically from reality. The "music business" became another example of this. Things happened fast in my life at that point, maybe too fast. All I can say is, if you think politics is dirty, man, try the music business for losing money, quite possibly your soul and even a song. While it's true that I met and worked with some fantastic people, people who helped me through the maze of the music industry, people who helped me through my battles with my health and cancer, those who helped me connect with others, I also met people whom I would describe as shady, sneaky, deceptive, opportunistic, and underhanded.

Through writing and illustrating my children's book for Blue Cross Blue Shield, I met a friend who was solely interested in helping me out from simple sheer goodness. This person was one of the people without whom I would never have made a record or had some of the most memorable experiences of my life stemming from the music arena. She funded the recording of my song "Remission." I remember the day I wrote that song, thinking, "This is a good one." I was so excited about "Remission" that I quickly recorded a raw version of it on my cell and texted it to my friend and backer.

"Oh man, what do you think about the hook in this chorus?" I asked. And from there, it was on to the studio.

This song eventually garnered me some attention from a merchandising company, and now looking back, I truly believe these guys had one thing in mind, making money and not at all reaching people with my story and message.

Around this same time, a large national cancer organization also entered into the picture. They wanted me to sing "Remission" at one of their big events. However, my ol' buddies who did the merchandizing sent a cease-and-desist to this cancer organization, stopping me from performing at one of their biggest events. Why? Well, because a few months earlier, the merchandising folks had forced me to sign over the song to our newly formed LLC "or else." Was it because they saw an opportunity with my song and wanted in on it? No need for head-scratching here. As I recall it, I was told I needed to sign over the song "Remission" or they would move ahead with my very own project—without me!—a project I had put together on paper years earlier.

In the end, I did sign away the rights to "Remission"—yes, a stupid move, I know—but at the time I was having some health issues, most likely residual effects from medical procedures years earlier. And I was also feeling enormous pressure from this company and myself to make my project become a reality.

I eventually removed myself entirely from the project. The merchandising company simply plugged in another person's story into my project and moved forward with it. They created a website, and all sorts of merchandise went up for sale. I have to admit, it was weird logging on to a website based on an idea I had created and seeing someone else's story. However, shortly after, the site went down. Last I checked, I couldn't find the site, and I couldn't find any merchandise.

Could there be a silver lining in the loss of a song and such a crappy experience? Well, yes, I ended up writing another song in place of "Remission." It's the song "Survivors Survive" I mentioned. To this day I've performed it at countless rallies across the nation. The song was used on #WorldCancerDay in 2015 and is now played for survivors all over the world.

Then there was my song "Where Hope Lives" that I wrote and recorded for the American Cancer Society Winn Dixie Hope Lodge. I recorded it for free and performed it at the ACS's "Coaches vs. Cancer" event in Atlanta, Georgia. It was an awesome night, one of my best ever.

Shortly after that performance, I moved from the grind of being a musician to the grind of working in a corporation. I remember sitting at my desk one day when my cell phone rang.

"Ryan, how are you?" the lady on the other end of the phone asked.

She was a former contact I had worked with before. And, though I had not heard from her in a while, she had listened to my song, "Where Hope Lives," and was interested in using it.

"Everybody here loves your song 'Where Hope Lives,'" she told me. "How would you feel about our organization using it in a commercial?"

"Of course!" I said and thought, *How great would this be?*

But then I realized I needed to think her offer through more carefully. When I did, I found a few small problems with the deal. For one, there was no money in it for me, and when I asked if I could be in the commercial, well, too late, they had already made the thing. So in return, I was offered a PR campaign, the universal currency of those who don't wish to pay an upcoming artist in good old green. If you are any kind of performing musician, you've of course heard the "It will get you exposure!" line.

It can be argued that flattery and exposure are great forms of currency, but they don't pay the bills. So how do you think this story played out? Call me a bad businessman, and I might agree, but I didn't get paid and that organization got their commercial. Did you ever hear about this or me? No? Well, that may be because I never got that whole PR thing I was promised.

Honestly, though, I was pleased when it came to the sum total of things. Later, several other songs of mine would be licensed, and I would be paid for them. Though life comes with many disappointments, I know I will always be a musician. You might say I survived the music industry, as well as cancer. And looking back, I like to think that perhaps a few people heard the lyrics to my song "Where Hope Lives" and found a little hope.

Chapter 4

The Country, the Business, and That Badass Corvette

*Life is to be lived, not controlled; and humanity is won by
continuing to play in the face of certain defeat.*
–Ralph Ellison

By the time my brother and I were enrolled in public school, I had been treated for cancer twice. Because my mom worked at the private Christian school we had been going to, she got a discount on tuition. But by the time I was nine, and thankfully back in school after my second round of treatments, my mom was no longer working at that school and my parents couldn't afford the tuition for Jason and me. But my mom and dad were happy to get us into the public school, as it was a good school. And I was glad to be back among kids my age, going to classes, being a kid again.

This exciting turn of events meant that this new school Jason and I would attend had big, new playgrounds, a huge new basketball court, and even some new kids. I even started there as a semipopular kid—imagine that! It was like a new beginning after I was cured (that second time), and at nine years old, believe me, even the smallest positive changes can make a world of difference.

I was in sixth grade, my last year of public grammar school, when I was hit by cancer a third time. By that time, though—weird as this might seem—cancer was kind of just life for me. I had gone through two rounds of cancer, treatment, and recovery by the age of eleven, and even though I had emerged cancer-free each time after going through treatment, I never felt normal by the usual standards for a kid my age. It was like I had two legs, eyes, ears, and, yes, cancer.

For my mother, well, my cancer diagnosis was a little too familiar:

Nothing is harder than finding out the first time that your child is sick with cancer; it is absolutely horrifically life changing in a way you can never imagine. But in a way I was just as devastated when I got the news again; Ryan has cancer, not once, not twice, but at that point three times. There is no way you are prepared for it, no matter what you've faced before. Each time Ryan presented with cancer, I was torn up. You are supposed to be able to protect your children, but in this case, there's nothing a parent can do other than make sure you get to the treatments and be as supportive, positive, and loving as you know your child needs you to be.

It's funny (funny strange, not funny "haha") when I think back on it now, how many times people would ask me how I felt. I knew that they were judging me by the standard of somebody who wasn't sick almost every day of his life, not somebody who always felt a little "off" even on his best days. Not somebody who was exhausted by treatments and procedures and worry. Not somebody whose week could have as easily meant a run to the store as a few runs back and forth to the hospital. Not somebody who had been introduced to sounds and smells that not even most adults ever become familiar with. No, "normal" for me was by no means the normal everybody else knew.

Actually, a year earlier, I had gone back to the hospital because I had developed an adhesion in my intestine. It all started with me sick, sitting on my couch, covered in a blanket, suffering terrible stomach cramps. I was watching an '80s movie, *Indiana Jones and the Temple of Doom*, the one with that kid, Short Round, screaming "Dr. Jones! Dr. Jones!" As often happened to me, the rest of the neighborhood was up to its usual that day—street football games, kids running around without a care in the world—while I was stuck inside. My dad thought I was just constipated and had me drink a big bottle of prune juice. He really did have an aversion to going to the hospital. The last thing he wanted to do was to admit that what was going on with me was anything serious (I can't blame him). But the prune juice didn't work. In fact, I had to be put into a cold tub to bring down my fever. I ended up getting sicker, throwing up all the prune juice in the tub (sorry, but it's true) and being rushed to the ER at the Medical Center in Columbus, Georgia. From there, they decided to do surgery.

It was hell. The adhesion was scar tissue from a previous surgery that wrapped around my intestine and cut off anything flowing through my intestine. After you are treated for cancer, you are left with a whole bunch of long-lasting complications that can result from getting "cured"; this was just one of them. You might not have the disease anymore, could be years from your last treatment, but this doesn't mean you still might not suffer complications, even ones that could be life-threatening.

At eleven years old, I was facing sixth grade with as much energy as my body could muster, including street football games, collecting baseball cards, and trading them. Ninety-nine per cent of that summoned energy was spent on my new obsession... skateboarding.

Woefully skinny and small at just a smidgen over seventy pounds, I was still pretty much the target for bigger kids who would try to push me around, although I was always pushing back. But the saving grace of my world, something where my size and weight were actually an advantage, was "catching air" with my friends as much as I could. I was a fan of a group of popular skateboarders called the "Bones Brigade," who took their name from the unique whiteness of the wheels their boards sported. I'd pour over *Thrasher* magazine, featuring pictures of the Bones Brigade, who would perform tricks that defied the laws of physics.

To the constant annoyance of our neighbors, my brother Jason and I, along with our friend Chris and his friend Steve, would jump the homemade ramps we laid out on our street. We bought or used old plywood and 2x4's to build those ramps, with Chris eventually acquiring a wooden "quarter pipe" for a lot of our skateboard tricks. Rumors of any other neighborhood area with a makeshift natural ramp or a cool surface would prompt exploratory excursions where we'd hopefully find ourselves speeding faster or reaching higher. As I think back to one of our most favorite spots on Primrose Road near our house, I realize my mom would have undoubtedly had a heart attack if she would have witnessed me flying down that high hill.

I was the youngest in our group, and often I'd be a little nervous to jump off some of these huge ramps like the older guys, but I'd make myself do it. My seventy pounds was mostly bones, but I'd hear my brother yell encouragement like: "Come on, Ryan. It's your turn, man. Get going fast so you can catch some air!"

Off I'd go. Although I can count one broken leg in the bunch (thankfully not mine; that's all I would have needed, right?), I guess you could say we had our own *Broken* Bones brigade, a wacky, air-jumping bunch. Moving like that, with speed and antigravity skill, made me forget—even for an ever-so-brief time—all the crap that had gone down in my short life. Yes, Jason often said, "Did you see how fast I was going? You may jump higher than me on the ramp, but I don't think you skate faster!" Still, I knew I flew on my board. When the Hodgkin's came calling that year, I knew that not only would the treatments begin again (oh, lucky me) but I'd miss school and not hang out with my friends as much. But what bothered me most was that my boarding would be halted. But Dad came to my rescue and decided to buy me a new board.

I chose a Lance Mountain model, the very board used by Lance Mountain of the Bones Brigade. As I've told you, many of my memories have been lost or splintered over time via chemo brain. But I do distinctly remember walking into OJ's skateboard showroom the very day I was diagnosed for the third time with cancer, drooling over the boards hanging the full width and height of the wall before my dad and me. And I remember Dad saying, "Just get the one you want."

I gave him my "for real?" look, stunned into speechlessness. We left the shop, me on my way to building my dream board.

I completely decked the thing out; it sported the coolest trucks and wheels and was so bad I almost didn't want to use it. The thought of getting home after a chemo treatment and being able to take that board out got me through some tough times that year, I can tell you. It wasn't hell 24/7. Plenty of kids came over, and the girl next door was really sweet. She was quite cute, actually; I secretly had a crush on her, and she'd turn out to be the first girl I ever kissed (one of my big-time secrets, among others that will be revealed in this book!). She even made me one of the bracelets that were all the rage at the time.

One of the brightest spots in my life were the times I went with my family to "the country," as I've mentioned briefly already. This meant we went out to where my cousins and their parents, my Aunt Nancy and Uncle Mike, lived, way out on their farm in Cataula, Georgia. The place was a treasure trove of delights for a kid, especially someone like me who loved the outdoors and was always starving to get out, to get sweaty and get plenty dirty after too much time in the sterile environments of hospitals or spending too many days recuperating inside my house. There were acres of green pastures, two lakes for fishing, woods to explore, plenty of spots to set up pretend army camps, and spacious areas to practice my BB gun shooting. My two cousins never seemed to tire of living there, always ready for any kind of adventure, from climbing trees to catching catfish.

That farm also had many animals; Noah himself would have been jealous. My dad's sister, my Aunt Nancy, loved animals, and she'd take anything in, from rabbits, cattle, cats, chickens, you name it. Even a squirrel came to stay, although my aunt didn't capture or invite him. I guess he just set up residency. The word among the critters in that area had to have been that my aunt and uncle's farm was a great place to be if you had four legs.

Luckily, I got to visit the country for about a week at a time. There was no Snapchat then. Imagine an eleven-year-old boy out there with nothing else to do but explore, not communicating with anyone except for who came by to walk through the woods with me. Those green pastures and all those chittering animals were all I could ever have wanted.

I threw back many of the fish I caught in the lakes at my aunt and uncle's farm, but I could never throw away the memories I have of those sunshiney days in that magical place.

I also have great memories of my fantastically loving sets of grandparents on both sides. Both my mom's mom and dad, and my dad's parents were wonderfully warm people, especially showering me with their affections given my particular obstacles growing up. Often when I didn't go to school, deep in the throes of getting over my latest round of treatments, or just not feeling up to going anywhere in public, I'd stay with either pair.

My mom's parents, whom I called Granny and Granddaddy, owned a small printing business, and I can remember staying with them during some school days while my mom and dad worked. Most of the time while staying at "the business," as we called it, Granny would set me up a cot to sleep on in between working on my own "projects."

Granny was a small, soft-spoken woman who was always a tad bit nervous. She wanted everything and everyone to be okay. It was a sweet quality I realize now, but she did walk around a little jumpy. While at the business, Granny always made sure I had plenty of food, snacks, drinks, more food, and a daily dose of the Bible. Yes, it was the typical spoiling of a grandchild, and I came to love the treatment.

Those "projects" of mine? Well, Granny set me up to work on my first series of books. They were more like pamphlets, always about aliens for some strange reason, which doesn't surprise me so much, because to this day I'm still totally fascinated by aliens. The first book I wrote was *The Mornz*, and the second book was named *Maro the Martian*. I know these first forays into publishing sound utterly ridiculous, and they were probably chemo-induced, but it was a thrill to be able to stretch my imagination this way, do some real work as I saw it at the time, alongside my grandparents' printing and publishing.

Sometimes I'd even do a little work to make some money. God knows I needed to feed my habit... earn money for more G.I. Joe men, baseball cards, fishing lures, or Transformers. So I'd help my granny put together the books they made.

While staying at the business, my Granddaddy Goodlett would talk to me about fishing, life, my brother, the Bible, and a whole host of other things. And my grandmother, "Granny" or "Rubes," as my brother called her, would talk to us about what my granddaddy should not be talking to me about: girls, gossip, and mythical tales.

"Oh, your granddaddy is making that up," Granny would say to me. "Stop it, Jimmy. You know that's not true," she'd scold him.

Granddaddy would look at me and smile as Granny continued to lecture him. Man, I loved those two and being smack dab in the middle of their obvious affection for one another.

Often while working or sleeping on the cot in a tiny office, I could hear printing presses running, Granny trying to drum up some business on the phone, and the commotion of a typical day. I'd hear my granddaddy whistling (he did this a lot) in between answering the phone: "This is Jim, how can I help you?" All of this, the noise and the craziness of their business, was comforting, a reminder for me that there was life in motion outside of chemo, radiation, surgery, and anxiety.

The business was a pretty cool place for a kid. I will always remember the people that came in and out: Mary, Willie, Billy, and of course Rubes and Jim. What a great bunch of characters.

Now my dad's parents, Bamba and Granddaddy Hamner, also played a major role in my life. All the grandkids loved going to their house. Heck, everyone in the family did; this is where the pool was.

I'll splash into telling you about that in a second (sorry, couldn't avoid that pun), but I do want to impress upon you how all my grandparents were always trying to help me put on weight, the weight I had lost from chemo. In fact, Granddaddy Hamner began a little program where he would pay me a dollar for every pound I gained. That was good money to me then, so I ate like a boss.

From both sides of the family, I was fed London broil, bacon, eggs, and grits at any time of the day. I had pound cake, BLTs, tuna salad, peanut butter and jelly, Skor bars, and even the notorious Spam. My grandfathers were especially determined I'd get up to the healthy weight of a kid my age. We Southerners can eat, let me tell you!

Bamba and Granddaddy's house had TVs with HBO and Cinemax. They had an Atari (the PlayStation of my generation) with a game console that had a joystick with one button instead of a controller and two triggers and A, B, C, D, E, and F buttons. Can you imagine? This would be like describing the Stone Age to kids today. And they had that pool… with a slide!

I spent many days in my Bamba and Granddaddy's backyard, whether it was on a weekend with my family, aunts, uncles, and cousins at the pool, or during the week if I needed to be home from school because I didn't feel well, had doctor's appointments, or just needed a break. Bamba and Grandaddy's backyard was on a double lot, and it wasn't just any backyard. My grandparents loved to plant flowers and be outside hard at work. There was always something for them to do in that big yard, something to make better, and their yard showed how much they loved being out there.

The backyard had paths through flower gardens, tall Georgia pine trees, miscellaneous plants and bushes throughout. From a kid's perspective, the backyard had a huge hill, and on one side of it sat a garden. My granddaddy and I would work in that garden, pulling weeds, tilling the soil, and my favorite, picking crops like cucumbers, tomatoes, and the best, of course, watermelons. Yes, much of the time I was sick from my treatments, but working hard out in that sunshine with all those fresh smells, sights, and sounds was the best cure for me.

"How are you liking school? Keeping those grades up?" my Granddaddy Hamner would ask as we worked. Other times he'd tell me a story from back when he was in Panama or Guam. I remember the scene vividly, Granddaddy in his work pants, an old flannel shirt, and one of his many mesh-style trucker hats sitting on his head.

Many Saturdays, while the family was at the pool, my grandparents would bring us watermelon from their garden. We'd then sit at the homemade white wooden table that sat between the garden and pool and eat our watermelon. At times like these, thoughts of chemotherapy and the coming nausea were temporarily tamed and silenced.

The pool was as fantastic as the garden, of course in a totally different way. This was where all the action for my family took place on any given summer weekend. Next to the pool was a mostly wooden rectangular-shaped building that we called the bathhouse. Inside this structure was a TV, kitchen, bathrooms, and a sofa to be lazy on — a cozy little place.

My grandparents' pool had a diving board and a slide that we all loved. My Granddaddy Hamner rarely would get into the pool, but he loved to sit in one of the chairs by the pool under an umbrella, watching us have fun. I get the feeling he sat there feeling proud of where he had come from, his kids, his grandchildren, and this spectacular yard he and my Bamba had built and that we all loved so much.

At home, my parents would merely have to say the words "Bamba's pool," and Jason and I would overflow with excitement, thinking and talking about nothing else until it was time to go there once again. I mean, all my family seemed to love spending time at the pool and being with Bamba and Granddaddy.

Sometimes, when I go back home, I drive down Flint Drive purposely just to go by my grandparents' old house. There is another house on the other lot now and nothing looks the same, but I can recall all those good times… even with my bad memory. Many times, especially when I drive by, I wish so bad I could just go back for one more swim with my family — and one more afternoon working in that garden — and get one more glimpse of that proud look on my granddaddy's face.

It is true, you never know how much you miss something until it's gone; then you miss it a lot.

Treasures for me are the memories of planting the garden with my granddaddy, the smells of the garden earth when we'd pull the radishes and onions from the ground, the taste of the fresh garden tomatoes on the BLTs my Bamba would make for me. On a good day for me, I'd be helping with the grass cutting or car washing, and sometimes my granddaddy would take us to the lake to fish or to shop at the commissary.

One particular day, I wasn't feeling too great while at school, but Granddaddy Hamner knew just how to cheer me up. At the time, my granddaddy owned this fantastically cool '64 Corvette, which my brother now owns. (He tracked that car down a few years ago, paid the premium price, and hauled it back home for all of us in our family to enjoy even now.) All of us grandkids were always begging to go for a ride in that smokin' hot car, but it wasn't always possible for whatever reason; Granddaddy liked to keep that thing shiny and covered up.

Anyway, on this one school day when I felt sick as a dog, my granddaddy showed up in the Corvette to pick me up from school. My jaw dropped. This was total awesomeness!

"Granddaddy!" I exclaimed when I saw him.

"Get in, Ryan Q," he said with a smirk. He knew I loved riding in the Corvette. I asked him one time what that nickname meant, and he simply said, "Quick... it means you're quick, Ryan."

Standing there in my Duke Boys shirt at the front of the school, I opened the door to the Corvette and got in, feeling kind of like life in slow motion. You know, like I was a badass from some Hollywood movie—some cool tune playing, and me, slowly stepping into my granddaddy's Corvette. The only thing that could have made things cooler is if there were some sort of explosion as we drove off and if I were wearing a pair of sunglasses. As we drove away, I hoped that as many of my young female schoolmates as possible were watching me get into that car. No, I wasn't all that into girls yet at the ripe old age of ten, but still, I sensed that "chicks digging the ride" you are in was kinda cool.

Granddaddy Hamner steered us right onto the road right in front of the school, and I knew—and hoped—he wasn't going to pass up an opportunity to show me, and whoever was watching us, what a badass he still was. That is when the old guy put the pedal to the metal!

The floorboard quickly began to vibrate from the engine torque, and the next thing I knew, we were up to fifty miles per hour on old Edgewood Road. Let me tell you, that old car could move. And for a ten-year-old, fifty miles per hour was like 150 mph, especially driving in an area with a twenty-five mile-per-hour speed limit. I loved it.

That wasn't the end of what my granddaddy was getting up to with me and his car that day, though. He decided to hit the highway. I remember as clear as day watching my Granddaddy Hamner get the Corvette up to eighty miles per hour as we shot out onto the highway. You can believe I was watching the speedometer closely so I could go back and brag later about how fast I went. Man, what a guy my Granddaddy Hamner was.

Throughout the years of being sick, I had many surgeries, treatments, and infections. But I always looked forward to my grandparents coming to see me in the hospital. I can remember every time that I had a surgery or medical procedure, Bamba and Granddaddy and Granny and Granddaddy would come into my hospital room. They wouldn't frown. They would smile like nothing was going on.

Granddaddy Hamner would always say, "Ryan Q!" and grin.

All my grandparents would ask: "What do you want when you come back to your room?" As most kids do, I loved surprises, so I'd always ask for the all-important "goodie bag." That third time diagnosed, as much as any of the times before, I lived for what surprises those goodie bags would bring me. When I would return, I'd have two goodie bags. They'd have G.I. Joe men, parachute men, wax lips, Life Savers, baseball cards, and Big League Chew. And sometimes, they'd even throw in stuff I needed, like socks.

My grandparents helped make the hard times better times. They were always there. Thinking back on all of what they gave me, how they enriched my life, how they rose to those occasions when they all knew I was feeling awful (and had to be scared themselves over what I was going through), I realize I was pretty well blessed—Corvettes, BLTs, HBO, G.I. Joe men, books, Spam... but mostly their love.

You certainly miss people terribly when they are gone, and our grandparents, if we are lucky to have them at all during our growing-up years, are most likely going to die during our lifetimes. But even the deep pain of a loved one dying doesn't eclipse the love and warmth I have deep in my memory from what the wonderful older people in my life gave to me. That love will live as long as I do.

Chapter 5

Granddaddy Hamner and Me, Ryan "Q"

Any day above ground is a good day.
–Granddaddy Hamner

As I mentioned, 1994 was a bad year; Granddaddy Hamner died that year, and my world was torn apart. As far as medical details, my granddaddy had emphysema from many years of smoking. I can remember him many times struggling to breathe but still going about his business like nothing was wrong, doing everything any normal person would do. He still worked his garden and drove to his beach house in Panama City Beach, Florida, where my family would meet him and my Bamba sometimes. He was just living life in his usual determined, unique way, listening to no one, being his own man, loving life and his family.

Looking back, it's clear to me now what was going on right before my Granddaddy Hamner died. He had asked me to help him after school to clean up his belongings. This wasn't so unusual in and of itself, as I often worked side by side with my granddaddy in his garden and we were very close; I was crazy about the guy. But that year, when I was in the twelfth grade, I'd go over to my granddaddy's house to help him clean out the place. That project was lots of work but fun.

I got to hang out with my granddaddy and go through his military stuff, which was another fascination of mine. We came across things I never knew he had. He told me great stories, and I learned so much more about his life.

"Pick those papers up, Ryan. You know what those are? Those are declassified files from the military days," he'd say as I came upon a pile or two. Now whether or not Granddaddy Hamner was kidding, I still, to this day, don't know. And, to this day, I still don't much care.

I realize now that my granddaddy was getting things in order because he knew his time was running out. Of course, I had no clue about this aspect of the clean-up. All I knew was that I was hanging with this guy who I so adored, and we were having a great time. Really, how could things have been any better? This wasn't about me being sick, my granddaddy attempting to take my mind from my cancer or its treatments, spinning me to and fro with his 'Vette, being by the pool with him. This was just us working to go through this stuff and him regaling me with his memories over the items we would come upon.

As a matter of fact (don't judge me for being clueless, okay, I just wasn't considering his mortality at the time), after we cleaned out the attic, we laid out items on the dining room table, and my granddaddy invited family members to come and take what they wanted. I took Granddaddy's flannel shirt that I used to see him wear in the garden. That was valuable to me. I would later play some of my first gigs wearing that shirt. Everybody else came and took things too. Again, hindsight is 20/20, and if anybody else had any clue what was really happening, nobody let on. At least nobody let on to me.

My Granddaddy Hamner was one of the most important men in my life. If you are lucky to know your grandparents in your lifetime and you especially take to one or any of them, the particular bond that can grow spanning generations can be something quite special. And though, yes, I loved all my grandparents—you have read they were all extraordinary people in my life and showered me with love—my Granddaddy Hamner was da man, numero uno with me!

The guy was a war hero, a self-made man, a tough guy, a mentor, unshakable in his convictions and in how he carried himself, a man who loved his family to the depth of his soul. He was merely one-of-a-kind, the type of man that we rarely see, especially these days.

Sitting on the couch in our living room one night, I heard my dad say to the person on the phone, "I'm going to have to let you go, my father is in the hospital, and this may be the last time we get to see him."

I didn't know who my dad was speaking to on the phone. It was in the afternoon, and I had just come home from school. I knew things were bad with my granddaddy, but I couldn't accept where it all seemed to be headed. How had we gotten here so fast, from me helping to clean out the attic to this horrible reality? Looking back, one of the oddest things about that moment was how calmly my dad talked to the caller on the other end of the phone about what I suddenly realized—his dad was dying.

Then again, what else could he do? This was all happening, my Granddaddy Hamner was slipping away, and nobody could do a thing about it.

After my dad hung up the phone, he moved deliberately throughout the house, locking doors, and turning off lights.

"Come on, let's go see Granddaddy," he said.

I felt sick and nervous.

As we headed to the hospital, I realized I was on the other end of things now. For all my life, my granddaddy had been the one standing at the foot of the bed, cheering me on. Now it would be me standing at the foot of his bed, cheering him on. I didn't have a plan as to what to do or say, though; I was totally unprepared for this. Granddaddy Hamner had never been unprepared when he visited me.

I remember walking onto the floor of the hospital and being hit with too many sense memories. I had hoped I'd never have to be reminded of these things: those particular smells, the hum and other weird noises the hospital equipment made, even the look of the place. It was confusing as much as it was all too familiar being there. Here I was, back in a hospital, in an ICU in fact, but I was healthy; I was the one visiting. Man, the world was upside down right then, I can tell you that!

We reached my granddaddy's room, and I saw him before he saw me. He was behind a sliding glass door, swollen, wearing an oxygen mask and lying in his hospital bed. This definitely wasn't how I was used to seeing this man, the same man who could work all day in the yard, fix anything, and cheer me up when I was at my worst. My granddaddy was strong. This didn't add up. Surprisingly, as I walked into his room, he smiled, like he always did.

"Ryan Q," he said as he held up his hand and reached for mine.

I walked over, reached up, and squeezed his hand. I held back my tears. Even though he was the one in bad shape, Granddaddy Hamner was still the one holding me up, with the squeeze of my hand and a smile. That part was still the same.

This is the last profound memory I have of seeing my granddaddy alive. He died shortly after Dad and I visited him in the hospital that day.

My Granddaddy Hamner's death hit me like a ton of bricks... make that two tons. Even with all I had gone through in my life, how many times I had flittered and flirted around death, my own or the many kids I saw undergoing treatment with me, this pain of losing this man was like nothing I had ever experienced. I was done in, wrung up over and out. Death had come to pluck one of the greatest men from the planet, and I was utterly devastated. I still am, in a way.

So, I turned to music again, and that's when I wrote "So Soon."

I'm not exactly sure, even to this day, how to put my love for Granddaddy Hamner into words. Indeed, a quick chapter in a book won't do the man justice. They say time heals all wounds, and yes, over the passing of years I have come to settle my mind and heart over my granddaddy not being around anymore. I miss the man every day, but you know how it is, even with those people you grieve over so profoundly, the stuff of life intrudes, and somehow you manage to get on with your day.

My Granddaddy Hamner lives in my heart, and that's about the best tribute you can give to anybody. I am better having known and having been loved by him in ways I will never truly ever be able to measure. The people who truly matter, who make the deepest impact, who contribute the most in making you who you are just by being who they were, never leave us. I'll probably start crying if I reread what I just wrote in this chapter, but it won't be tears of sadness; it will be tears of great joy for having had Granddaddy Hamner in my life.

Chapter 6

The Devil's Food Cake

If you learn from defeat, you haven't really lost.

–Zig Ziglar

In 1997, at the ripe old of age of twenty-one, I had my last occurrence of Hodgkin's lymphoma. Suddenly I was back on the same old routine from years ago—get on the road early in the morning a couple of times a week, stop by McDonald's, and then head on up to Emory in Atlanta for chemotherapy. G.I. Joe men weren't part of the routine this time. I was too old for them... though not too old for cancer, it seemed.

Already too well acquainted with this dadgum cancer from my three times previous, for this fourth and final occurrence (trust me, I'm not having it again!), we decided to go with the nuclear option, a bone marrow transplant. It would turn out to be the final nail in the coffin for my disease.

Now you can google all you want to about bone marrow transplants and what to expect, but I'm here to tell you, you can never prepare yourself for one. I'm not just talking about pain and discomfort. I'm also talking about the sheer craziness that goes along with having that procedure and how it affects your head—all part of "surviving," which I am coming to.

In 1988, the third episode of chemotherapy made me feel horrible. I mean, it's not like I expected that this orange, chemically smelling stuff that was burning my veins would make me feel like a rock star, but chemo my third time physically wrecked me in a way I could never have dreamed. I would get so sick after treatments sometimes that I thought I would never stop vomiting. But for this last time, in 1997, the "times they were a-changin'," as Bobby D. says. I would only have a few rounds of chemo before the transplant, but chemotherapy was a lot different in 1997 than it was in the 80s. (Heck, it's a lot different now than it was in '97.) And man, did this mess me up, but not like you may think.

Dreading nausea, I was rattled, anxious, nervous… and really ticked off about having to go through all this again! With my family, I waited in the waiting room of the chemo clinic at Emory's Winship Cancer Institute, all of us trying to talk, laugh, downplay, and distract ourselves from what we were there for—the chemo again. I remember looking around the waiting room at the different patients there. I wondered of course what their prognoses were and where they were from, the same as I had when I was a kid. All of us in that room had stopped our day-to-day lives for this, our cancer affecting where we could go, what we could eat, who we could be around, how we slept, and about a thousand other things a healthy person would never think about.

I really hated this, and I knew everybody else waiting with me in that room, the patients as well as their family members, hated it as much as me. Don't think for a moment, though, that misery loves company. Any one of us would have been out the door right quick if somebody had come in and told us our diagnosis was wrong, that we were cancer-free. Sorry, but I'm speaking the truth here. We are indeed all sympathetic to one another, caregivers and cancer patients both. But give me the chance then, or anytime I had cancer, and I would have spun out of a treatment room and never looked back.

Well, OK, maybe I do look back… this book is a result of that, as is my music and writing career, which is centered around surviving. But you get my point. I DID NOT WANT TO BE GOING THROUGH TREATMENT AGAIN.

When my name was called for chemo, it felt like the last time I had been there. Talk about the crappiest kind of déjà vu. I stood slowly and managed that terrible walk I had done so many times before. I walked back to the chemo room, imagining CJ or Miss Sydney greeting me. How I would have loved to be welcomed by their warmth and smiles. As I walked into the main area of the chemo room, which had a much fresher, newer look than my other clinic, I teared up. I tried to hold my emotions in check, but I couldn't. My eyeballs had a mind of their own, and I started crying.

The nurse led me to my chair and gave me the verbal tour, telling me where the restroom was and how to use the remote control for the TV. She was trying to make me feel at home, but we all knew this was not home, although the staff were great people.

They cleaned and "accessed" my port with a small needle thingy (yes, that's the medical term). My port was a little round disc right below the skin on my chest, connected to my carotid artery. These were new things, ports. They saved the veins on people's hands that would often become weakened and ultimately destroyed by chemotherapy. It was a nice invention, I thought, but heck, my veins had already become faint little green lines by then. My veins were so bad in my right arm that little kids used to comment on them. That's the real test to see if you really have a noticeable physical flaw on your body—big nose, skinny legs, that birthmark you always try to cover up. If you ever wonder whether what you are worrying about is noticeable, ask a kid. They will gladly tell you what is wrong with how you look. Even if you don't ask, they often still gladly tell you.

"Your arm looks like it has green worms in it."

"Yes, I know," I'd reply. "I got them from saying rude comments to adults when I was about your age."

After flushing some saline through the port, it was time. No sign of CJ. I sure would have liked to have been holding an army man right then that I had snatched off of Miss Sydney's cart. Yeah, I know I was twenty-one, but I was hurting deep inside. I REALLY did not want to be here.

How about a ShowBiz run afterward?

My mom, my dad, and I all sat anxiously waiting. I'm sure we were all thinking the same thing: "How bad is this going to be?"

The nurse began the chemo drip, and we continued our wait. A few moments later, she showed up with something in a syringe. Hmmm, was it just another saline flush or an antinausea medication like I'd been given in the past?

"You probably didn't have this during your last treatments; it's fairly new. It will fix you right up," said the nurse.

An hour went by, and I felt nothing. No nausea, nothing. Not even a stomach gurgle. Instead, I was starting to get real friendly with everyone in the room and was actually feeling *hungry.*

At the two-hour mark, I found myself eating a turkey sandwich and flirting with the girl across from me, who I would later date, briefly.

Could this be happening? I'm having chemo, feeling half drunk, and eating a turkey sandwich while talking to a cute girl? This was nuts!

The treatment still took as long as it always did, though. My parents would pass the time by reading books and magazines, watching the news, going for walks, heading down to the cafeteria. And this time they could even let me know when they were headed there. Heck, this time they even ate right in front of me.

During my earlier treatments, the sight, smell, or even thought of food could "bring up" the worst in me. In the early years, my poor parents had to manage all sorts of clandestine operations to get a friggin' sandwich. I remember thinking as a kid that my parents would never get to eat again. I never saw them with any food. I eventually figured out that they weren't rushing out of the room to make five or so critical phone calls every day. They were hungry, and they were headed out to grab some food.

As my treatment that day came to an end, a nurse cleaned up the port, threw away the needles, and sent us on our way for a few days. I was pretty happy it had all gone so well. When we got home that night, I was a bit tired and had a slight headache, but nothing too crazy. I certainly was not throwing my guts up continually, didn't need a cold washrag on my head. None of that. I was in the clear.

The next day, I woke up after sleeping hard and thought, "Hey, I'm fine. This is going to be easy stuff." My attitude was perfect. Nothing in my life was going to change because of treatment this time. It was almost a decade later now that I was going through this again, and things had changed big time! I was going to be the dude from the movie *Unbreakable*, although I couldn't run that well or hold wooden beams over my head.

I ate some breakfast (I ate breakfast!), put on my gym clothes, and headed to go work out. It was leg day; I was going to do squats, leg curls, that sort of thing. I was going to work out as hard as I always did. Why not? I felt great.

When I got to the gym and walked inside, my brother and friends were all eager to find out how I was feeling and how things were going. They knew of my history and what I was going through. I was so thrilled to be at the gym, thinking it would be at least a year and a half or more before I would be able to go back due to treatment. Man, was I ever ready to get started.

I began squatting. I did a warm-up set, and all was good. I felt great. I looked around the gym and thought, nothing is changing, it's all truly the same. I did another warm-up set, and I still felt good. So then I moved on to the sets where I did even heavier weights, heavy for me anyway. It was the slow motion, Hollywood movie thing again. I was jamming to workout tunes and trying to get after it.

I did approximately three more sets and then, BAM! It hit me. Out of nowhere, I started sweating; my stomach got miserably sick. I was getting dizzy, fast, and I was suddenly totally exhausted. I was also a bit panicky and confused. I mean, I had woken up feeling great. I had even eaten that turkey sandwich during chemo and flirted. I had had breakfast this morning. What the heck was going on?

I couldn't finish my workout. I quickly grabbed my bag and headed home. I was beat and sick. I could just hear my mom saying, "You shouldn't have pushed yourself like that."

When I got home, I went straight to bed and slept the rest of the day. I woke up briefly to my mom saying, "Ryan... Ryan... You need to take your meds," as she gave me a glass of water and a few pills. Then it was back to sleep. Even though I slept all day, I never felt rested. These new antinausea meds had pulled one over on me. I didn't throw up from the chemo. The drugs had worked well, in fact better than anything I had ever had or could ever dream, but ironically they had given me a false sense of security. The chemo still hit, and it hit hard! Well-played, chemo. Well played.

The next morning I was awakened and greeted by pain and exhaustion. Major pain. My whole body, but especially my legs, were aching (no surprise, huh?), tight, and most of all useless. I imagine if I were to be thrown out of my granddaddy's Corvette going eighty miles an hour that I might have felt the same way. What had I done?

What had happened was that those new antinausea drugs had made me feel so good that I was fooled into thinking I could work out as usual. But chemo is chemo and will drain you. This was a cautionary lesson for me to learn then, as well as something I know cancer survivors feel all the time. Even though there are wonderful new therapies and drugs out there for all kinds of serious diseases, current treatments and procedures can still kick your butt. Be careful, as even a few years ago what someone has gone through can be drastically different (and usually better) but you should always work out slowly until you know what to expect.

I won't take you through all of the steps before my bone marrow transplant. In a nutshell, I took a drug that made my body produce some cells that would be frozen through a process known as *hemapheresis*. Then I was on my way. I remember arriving at the hospital and checking in for the transplant. I have no idea why, but I was excited; maybe it was the Marinol (an antinausea drug that also could leave you high as if you had ingested a good amount of THC). I don't know why exactly, but I was ready. I was also determined not to let this procedure beat me into the ground. So I actually brought weights. Yep. I brought five-pound weights. You know those kinds that you get at Walmart that are coated in rubber or whatever? The type that can barely tone up an older woman's underarms? I had those.

When I arrived in my room, with all of my belongings, I was greeted by my nurse.

"Hi, I'm Gale. We're going to become great friends over the next couple of weeks. I need to lay out the rules for you so we can keep you healthy. What's this? Are you going to be playing me some songs on your guitar," she said with a smirk.

Gale and all the nurses I knew during my transplant would become like family before it was all said and done. They were great people. Actually, they were all too friendly up there to be putting new bone marrow into people. This made me suspicious. I didn't ask questions, though.

From here, I have to say, my memory gets foggy. It gets hazy, gray, clouded, unclear, fuzzy, and muddy. Maybe I was abducted or something. I have no idea, but I only remember bits and pieces. I have mentioned the term "chemo brain" before, but it's a real condition. Your head gets fuzzy from that poison they are putting into you. Sometimes it's short-term memory loss; sometimes you lose memories forever. I'd forget everything at times, or wait, did I? I remember once thinking that I was going to have to redo college, which might not be a bad idea, come to think of it. So let me just tell you, my memory got bad. I could only remember bits and pieces... and this would plague me for the long term.

One of the crucial pieces of a bone marrow transplant is to kill your current bone marrow. I know, it sounds violent, right? Well, they did it anyway. To accomplish this, I was given massive amounts of chemo, and I vomited massive amounts of, well, whatever. I got sick,

sick, and sick as a rabid animal. I also cussed, pressed my nurse call button repeatedly for meds, was moody as heck, and needed more meds. I wanted to break things but didn't have the energy and often forgot what I wanted to break. That's a frustrating combination.

I don't remember what was said before it all started. I don't remember if my nurse Jennifer or my nurse Gale administered the chemo, but I surely remember the effects of it all.

One evening I woke up and I could tell that I had slept for a long time and that I was miserably sick. I would vomit repeatedly and strain so hard I thought the vessels in my eyes would burst. It seemed never ending.

With the tissue-paper-like memory I have, many of these times have no color, depth, or feeling. It's more like the feeling of being surrounded by a grayish, cloudy, freezing day that I can walk into but not grab many pieces of the memories. I can recall brief snippets in my head of one of the nurses coming into my room to give me meds, me asking for the throw-up pan, or my mom wiping my mouth. Looking back, it's like I had the mute button on for the world around me. These were hard times.

I remember some of the nurse's names, Jennifer and Gale of course, but the rest are a blank. I forget who else was there. Jennifer is the nurse who pumped my new bone marrow into my IV. I remember that day clearly, September 22, 1998. I also have a picture that proves that Jennifer did pump the stuff.

I had what's called an "autologous" bone marrow transplant. Essentially, autologous is where your bone marrow is returned to you.

Now that part, actually "receiving the bone marrow," wasn't all that bad. However, fast forward a few days later, and I felt like I had fallen off a bike onto hard pavement and landed on my man parts. My most intimate of areas as well as under my arms became very raw, a weird and painful side effect of the procedure. Pain, severe pain. Pain like you have never felt. Yeah, good times.

I dozed back and forth through sleep and blurriness. Then one day, something I never thought would happen, well, happened. I mean, it was so bizarre that at first, I thought I was just in one of those half real-world, half delusional states.

Early every morning the doctors would make their rounds from patient to patient, and when they did, they had several students, residents or whomever, accompanying them. You would hear the light knock at your door, and then in walked the whole crew. They didn't wait for a yes or a no. It was just a notification knock to say, "Hey buddy; we are coming in. Aren't you thrilled?"

One particular doctor who came by always did the same thing: knock, enter and say, "Good morning. How are you?" then give the students a debriefing on me, my case, what stage of the transplant I was in, along with a bunch of medical stuff that you'd have to be in medical school to understand. I became somewhat of a lab rat for the class.

Now, keep in mind, I'm just waking up early in the morning. I'm on a pain pump, and a huge list of unpronounceable, barely google-able medications, and doctors and strangers just walk in on me, some of these new doctors only slightly older than me. They are all looking dead at me, and some of the ladies were kind of attractive.

So the doctor then asks me, as he is checking out the damage down below my personal Mason/Dixon line, if the "class" can take a look. Yes, the class that includes the attractive college-aged women. Well, thinking back, I was drugged out of my mind, so we weren't playing a fair game here. In any other circumstance, I would have refused... or demanded to be taken out for dinner first. "Sure. Go for it," I said.

Before I could get the words out of my mouth, the doctor had pulled the covers back for everyone to see... well... me. It was like I was in the Bodies Exhibit. Luckily this was during a time when no cam phones were available, not that anyone would have wanted a picture. Ah, the things we do for science.

Following my transplant, there were many days where I was lying in my hospital bed in a room that smelled way too clean. You know, that hospital, "the janitor just left" type of clean? I was in my boring, bland hospital gown, bald and spaced out with the TV going on and on about who knows. By this point, the TV shows and commercials all blended, and so did the days of the week. I often would wake up with some late-night infomercial running or with the strange desire to order some special chef knives or the Slap Chop.

My mom was sitting in a chair in the corner of the room, passing the time reading her magazines and books that she had probably read twice already. Occasionally she'd take or make a phone call to a friend or family member, updating on how we were doing.

"Yeah, he's sitting up, watching TV, eating some dinner. Oh, some meatloaf, green beans, and mashed potatoes," I'd hear her report.

It was understandable that friends and family wanted to know if I was feeling well enough to eat, but for some reason, almost all of them wanted to know what I was eating.

Only a few days after receiving my new stem cells as a part of my bone marrow transplant, the pain meds started to kick in. Wow. As I mentioned, one strange side effect of the transplant was that the skin under my arms and "down below" would really hurt. Because of this, I was hooked up to a much-needed pain pump. So when I felt "the burn," I could hit a button, and pain meds would be delivered straight into my veins. I would then enter into my little world, my own, creative little world far, far away. I'm not at all advocating doing drugs. I'm telling my story and the effects of my medication, medication I was extremely happy to have.

Often, or most of the time, I would just ramble. Ramble, ramble, and "Ramble on!" before falling asleep. I can remember this to some degree, but there are also plenty of witnesses who experienced my drug-induced rambles at one time or another who probably have better recollections than I do.

During this one particular night of rambles, Justin, my cousin, came by. He came to see me during my stay in the hospital for my bone marrow transplant almost every night. He'd come to sit there with me and read a book. He'd bring me magazines to read and would tell jokes. He'd always entertain me. Err, maybe I entertained him.

On this night, I can specifically remember talking about utter nonsense. Words of any type just came pouring out my mouth.

Justin and my mom just sat there, reading their books. They'd look up occasionally to see just how far gone I was. Looking back, all I can think is, how did they keep a straight face? I mean, even I knew I was out of it. I remember ending this particular session of rambles by saying something to my cousin about evil and "devil's food cake." Beyond that, I remember nothing accurately, other than seeing the inside of my eyelids.

My cousin and my mom were always understanding and calm about my rambles. Most of the time they agreed, nodding. However, they seldom had anything to add. They just went along with what I said, like everything made perfect sense. Sometimes they even looked like they were learning something. I think they did this just to switch things up.

On this one night, though, I said something that was a little out of the ordinary, which means it was probably more "ordinary" than out of the ordinary for me at the time.

"When I get done up here, I think I'm going to do a book for kids with cancer," I said to my mom and cousin. I was serious. Not that they were mean or dismissive, but I'm sure they all thought this was just more ramble. However, this ramble came to life.

When I got out of the hospital in 1998, months later, I began working on my children's book. I called it, *You'll Be All Right, Buddy!*

You'll Be All Right, Buddy! was an educational storybook for kids with cancer. All of the characters in the book were named after people I met while going through my bone marrow transplant, or people who were right by my side. Okay, honestly, there may have been a few imaginary people in that book, but my intentions were good.

There was Shannon, my good friend from high school; Sam; Buddy, of course; George; and the list of names goes on. All great people.

It was pretty amazing how the book thing came to be. I started out drawing a few pictures while recovering from my transplant. I wrote a little storyline, and then I started pitching it to different companies. I didn't want money. I just wanted to get my book out. I figured that the short storybook could help out a few kids battling cancer.

And in 1999, Blue Cross Blue Shield published my book. Newspapers ran stories about me and the book. I got to travel and read to children, kids battling cancer. My music career took off from around the book, as I have told you. It was a great time. An example of the proverbial "turning lemons into lemonade." And what it would lead to was a dream come true.

On top of remembering more stuff than I could even imagine I forgot, I view things a little differently whenever I read or hear my mom's accounts—her perspective of me dealing with cancer, the therapy, or some of the situations we have been thrown into. Her view of the world around us at those times is an insight into what goes on in the life of someone caring for a loved one who is sick.

So, I will share a piece she wrote about one of those times not so long ago:

I watched the young man push the woman in the wheel-chair up the wide, long ramp where I stood with my son, waiting just inside the transportation door at the clinic. Through the walls of glass, we could see tire tracks through the mounds of snow covering the streets and the huge foun-tain; its glistening jets halted in midair. That Sunday after-noon in a February blizzard, life moved slowly, and pieces of conversation mixed with noise from the crowd waiting, walking, or wheeling past. Slower still was the young man pushing his passenger, weaving in then out of the way of walkers, steering clear of the small clusters of patients and workers.

"You warm enough, Bud?" I asked Ryan, who pulled his cap down, reminding me of the sweet time when he was a child. The chilled air blustered against our faces each time the doorman in his red coat opened the glass door to announce a shuttle to a nearby hotel or a taxi to the airport. Breathing in, I could taste the cold. Ryan stuffed his hands into his jacket pockets. "Yeah," he said, looking past the crowd around us and me. And then, I knew Ryan had caught his first glimpse of the pair I had been watching for several minutes.

As the two wheeled closer, we realized their swerving path had much to do with the impaired gait of the young man pushing the wheelchair, speaking to the woman in a lisping, slurred speech. And, the reason for the wheelchair became apparent—the woman, old enough to be the young man's mother, had lost both legs. We could hear bits of conversation between them and realized that their disappointment was in the restrooms behind us where there was no "family" facility. As they turned awkwardly and slowly to head back down the long ramp toward another option, Ryan looked to me and whispered, "Mom, no one should ever have to suffer that much grief."

To say that Ryan has had four occurrences of Hodgkin's lymphoma, the last requiring a bone marrow transplant and other things—their descriptions limited by words—cannot convey what life for us has been. To communicate those things requires the experience itself, something I would never choose for another. But, as ironic as it may seem, the sweetness in our moments of joy is sharpened to another point where words again limit understanding. And, at times such as those, I am conscious that my brain halts long enough for me to revel in that joy—to soak up just a moment that will never come again. It is up to us to "see" beyond what we look at—to see and be reminded of the "sweet times"; to see and know that there is hope in a procedure, in a protocol, in a plan; to see and watch the wonder in water, frozen and halted in midair; to see the kindness in the words from those around us—a friend, a doctor, or maybe, even a stranger; and to see and be compassionate toward those others who may be struggling to navigate within that "invisible world." For it is truly, as Henry David Thoreau wrote, "not what you look at that matters, it's what you see."

After my transplant, I slowly transitioned back into my life. This meant finishing up school, getting a job, hanging out with my friends again, doing the things I wasn't able to do in the past couple of years—just getting back to normal. This also included coping with side effects, short term and long, and generally beginning to live as a cancer survivor.

Chapter 7

"It Ain't About How Hard Ya Hit. . ."

My past has not defined me, destroyed me, deterred me, or
defeated me; it has only strengthened me.
–Steve Maraboli

When you live through trauma, when you survive things that you maybe shouldn't have, you can't help but be impacted—mentally, emotionally, and physically. People often ask me, "How did you do it?" Well, I'm definitely no expert on how to survive cancer. I got through it (four times, thank you very much!) but most of the time, I was just flying by the seat of my pants or running over the bumps in the macadam with my skateboard, metaphorically and to use an example from my childhood. I got through because I just kind of got through, although I am very happy I did.

Heck, sometimes I acted on instinct, other times I felt like I could have (should have) given up, still other times I had a bad attitude, and then at yet other times, I focused and chose to do what it took to make it, to survive.

One of those times was in 2006.

Shortly after going into ventricular tachycardia while having a heart infection, I found myself being transported from Columbus,

Georgia, to Atlanta, Georgia. There I was told by the doctor at St. Joseph's Hospital that I might not make it.

"Ryan, I just can't promise you and your family you'll make it through this one," the doctor said with an intense look.

My mom, dad, and girlfriend at the time all froze after the doctor's comments. The weird thing for me was, what he said didn't frighten me. This wasn't because I was and am some super tough guy. No. For whatever reason, at that moment, faced with imminent death, I decided to focus. I became determined to get through my trial. Despite the dire news, I set my mind to survive as I always had. Admittedly, living this time was on a whole new dangerous scale. My body had "upped the ante" to be sure for this go 'round, but I was determined.

I lay in the hospital bed, in that sterile room behind a sliding glass door directly in front of the nurses' station. Too many times had I been in this particular situation and position, looking out on the bustling world around me, at the comings and goings of the hospital, nurses and doctors arriving for their shift or leaving after a long day. Too often I lay like this in some cold bed, alone long after or before my visitors would be coming for the day, simply contemplating my life and my seeming smallness in it.

Humbling? Um, yeah!

My heart was weak, in and out of normal rhythms, and my temperature was through the roof. I was in ICU and had been for days. And even upon receiving the doctor's horrible message, what was the all-too-real truth, I chose to focus on a simple plan. I decided to pray and focus on my breathing, as my hope for life rested in these two factors alone.

In the end, I made it through.

Hey, survivor here!

Did my plan do the trick? For me, the simplicity of focusing both my thoughts and my breathing did the trick.

The Formula

I've always heard the sayings: "Believe in yourself," "Think positive," "Be strong," etc. These are platitudes people puke at you or post on their social media with the best of intentions (and if it's not up on some sort of social media portal, it isn't real, right?). But when you are in the trenches of the most challenging times of your life, like fighting cancer, simple feel-good statements such as these do little to help. Spirit-raising statements are one thing, but this is big-time life and death stuff we are talking about here.

Maybe directions of some sort would help? A little guidebook pamphlet you can keep tucked under your hospital pillow or read nightly on your Kindle?

I developed a formula that worked as my strategy to help me through. Feel free to use it, or customize it to fit your needs. I am revealing it here and now with the hope that it helps somebody. After all, the reason I wrote this whole book was in the hope that my story, and most importantly this chapter, would help many people.

First up in the formula:

Surround Yourself with Good People

Let's face it, we all have those people in our lives that we aren't crazy about, folks you normally wouldn't hang with, the last people you'd want in the old sinking life raft. (Hey, don't feel so bad; in most cases when you feel this way about somebody, they most likely feel the same about you.) Sometimes you don't even have definable reasons why you don't like these people... although sometimes, man, you definitely do! They may be negative, critical, or bring you grief in the way they look at the world. People with agendas, people who play the passive-aggressive game; heck, you know the type. They may even be in your family. You know, those folks you kind of have to love because they are blood, but really, you'd rather you didn't know them? Well, part of my formula, and yes, I know it's not so easy to do, is to put these people out of your life for a while or at least to limit contact with them until you are in a place where you can tolerate them... i.e., healthier, in remission, or even, well... after a few drinks.

Remember, I am speaking to those of us who are either battling cancer or have recently gotten through it—survivors one and all—even caregivers. These people can learn much from my formula, and especially from this first step. You have read about my wonderful family: cousins, aunts, and uncles, my two sets of grandparents, my brother, and my parents—how they supported me and never let me feel down. My dad refused to let me feel sorry for myself, always pointing out some other kid who had it worse. I appreciate the freedom I had during times of fun abandon with my Granddaddy

Hamner, those times at the pool and in the country with my family around me. My mom was and continues to be my rock, my number one fan, the person I know who most has my back in ways I could never dream. These people loved and still love me unconditionally. I was safe with them. I could feel and do feel their love for me in everything they do and say.

Instead of allowing in those people in your life that you really don't like—and granted when you are down and out it's not the easiest thing to regulate who comes to see you—but best as you can, surround yourself with good people, people who truly care about you and won't bring you down. Consider letting your most trusted people know who's "in" and who's "out," to help you limit time with those who wipe you out. Hang out with people who make you laugh, who you know genuinely listen to what you say, and most importantly, people who you can be yourself with.

Think of it this way. Even on your best cancer-free, healthy, happy day, who likes to associate with someone they don't like? But when weighed down with some sort of serious health concern, when keeping a positive mindset is all important, be doubly aware of hanging only with the most uplifting people in your life.

Second in the plan:

Get a Hobby

Crochet, raise blue crayfish (yeah, I actually have a blue crayfish), collect coins, go to yard sales, read, start a blog, collect salt and pep-per shakers off of eBay—it doesn't matter what hobby you choose.

Having a hobby or two can give you something to look forward to when you are going through cancer treatments, are worrying about a diagnosis or surgery, or even years later, when you are recovering from it all.

I had several hobbies I could enjoy while in the hospital and others I could do when I'd get outside, even for a short time. One of those hobbies was metal detecting (laugh all you want; I found silver) and the other was sorting through boxes of coins, looking for rare ones. I believe my medication brought on some level of myopic madness that allowed me to sit for hours going through tons of old pennies in an attempt to find that one rare coin that would make me rich. But hey, whatever, it was something I enjoyed and looked forward to.

The bottom line is to find an activity that makes you want to get out of bed every morning... when, God knows, you might not want to. There has to be more to life than waiting around for another cancer treatment or throwing up after your last one. Looking forward to that day when you might be able to get up and skateboard with your buddies once again, or learning a new jiu-jitsu throw, maybe just going down to the store and seeing what new issues of the magazines you usually collect have come in—all afford you golden opportunities of anticipation. Many a day I lay in bed, either at home, at the Ronald McDonald House, or in the hospital, with my mind freed of the discomfort my body was going through because it could wander and wonder over all I was looking forward to in the myriad of interests and hobbies I had.

What you shouldn't do, and I know you will be tempted as I was at times, is to give up on those hobbies because you are sick. Sure, I had to stop pursuing my martial arts training, but that didn't mean I stopped being interested in martial arts altogether. Treatments and hospital visits might take you away, at least physically, from what interests you, but don't let cancer take your hobbies and diversions away for the long run. Fight to stay in the race, and live for those activities as you do everything else.

And a note to the caregivers. There will come times that you might feel pretty dadgum selfish about needing to get out for a concert, a road trip, or to hang out with a good friend. But do these things: go out and live your life too. The person you are caring for will want you to keep alive those things that mean the world to you, to enjoy even the passing interests you have.

Another on the hit parade here is as important to mind as well as body:

Exercise

I don't want to take up space writing the same old generic info about exercise. I also don't want you to think that the only way to benefit from working out is by running five miles a day and having chiseled abs (although chiseled abs are kinda awesome). For me, exercising consistently has been one of the most important decisions I've ever made for all aspects of my health: mind, spirit, and body. I believe, and many doctors have eluded to the connection, that my physical activity and my survival fit hand in glove. To say it straight, exercise is so important to health that keeping up some sort of exercise routine should be a no-brainer.

Look, I've been through hell. You've read all about it in the previous sections of this book. But I've always done some form of exercise. So take it from me, even if you are sick, and I mean dragged out, run over, heavy-duty, life-threatening ill, you still can manage some routine for physical activity. Yes, please consult your doctor about an exercise routine (she might even recommend something), but working your body in any way possible will yield positive benefits. For example, during my bone marrow transplant in 1998, I kept three-pound dumbbells in my hospital room. I did small "workouts"… and I mean very small, sometimes even while in bed. This weight routine, such as it was, offered me two benefits. One, it made me feel like I had, well, exercised, and two, it gave me a "small win"—a feeling of accomplishment. Believe it or not, "small wins" are actually a thing. They give us that feeling of "Oh yes, I achieved something; I did it." They release those feel-good chemicals in the brain. And man, did I ever need to feel good during those times I was feeling so bad.

OK, this next step in my formula is a biggie but a more personal one:

Pray

Are you a believer? If you're not, well, that's OK, but I am. Yes, I'm the guy who drops the F-bomb when I'm frustrated—when I've felt awful, stressed, and worried, and yeah, at other times, too. But still,

I believe in a God that hears my prayers (even when my behavior isn't the best).

For me, being a Christian has emboldened my hope and my will. My belief pushes me ever onward, and at times, the real tough times, that God-led fight has made a significant difference. My spirituality—feeling that particular indefinable connection in my most dire times—has been critical. But aside from what, for many, is often dismissed as dogma, many studies are now showing that the power of prayer is real, that prayer truly affects the physical body. Studies conducted at Duke, Dartmouth, and Yale Universities show that people who didn't participate in religion were fourteen times more likely to die after heart surgery. Elderly people who rarely, if ever, attended church had a stroke rate double that of those who did.

Harold Koenig, MD, associate professor of medicine and psychiatry at Duke University and senior author of the *Handbook of Religion and Health*, says that those who are religious tend to be less depressed than others, and this can impact overall health.

For me, my faith hasn't been about simply attending a church and declaring my religion out loud, or about trying to live a perfect life (um, I guess I have to give that up, huh?). Instead, my faith is about having that direct line to call out to, to give me hope.

And another truly personal part of the plan:

Play It Again

Obviously, music has been and continues to be a huge part of my life. It's been a constant as I've suffered through cancer over the years.

I define myself as much a musician as anything else: songwriter, performer, guitar player, singer. Simply listening to music makes me feel good. I seek out those good feelings when I'm down, and to me, music is the cheapest, healthiest, and fastest way out of the dump. Music has often been that influence that has connected me with the hope I needed to get through. It was something that reached beyond the pains of adversity, like when I sat for countless times in that chemo chair as a kid, grabbing my old Walkman and listening to those songs my brother and I had recorded from the radio.

These Days Are Different Days

The phrase "surviving cancer," calling someone a cancer survivor, or even the word "survivorship," as it relates to cancer, has a different meaning these days from what it did years ago… and for the most part, these differences represent incredible advances in cancer care. When I first presented with cancer, having the disease meant certain death, terrible reactions from chemo treatments, many long procedures, etc. This was not so long ago, really—as recently as the eighties. But considering all the scientific advances we have seen in even the past five years, really, cancer care when I was a kid and cancer care now are, in many ways, almost unrecognizable.

These days, cancer and its treatment are discussed in our mainstream culture. Men as well as women are treated for breast cancer. Cases pop up all the time of someone boasting a decade of being cancer-free. Celebrities like Angelina Jolie are open about undergoing elective preventive surgery for a cancer. In addition, new drugs, alternative treatments, new and improved ways of detection, and google-able knowledge of the various types of cancer means that things are better for us all as new technologies bring us ever closer to cancer cures. Look, I'm not saying in any way, shape, or form that I'd want to experience cancer at the present time, as much as I didn't want to suffer from it growing up. But I feel that these days, cancer patients have a better chance at a good quality of life, fewer side effects from treatment, and a great chance at a more sturdy and true remission.

But, although surviving is great, as a former cancer patient, you still face challenges ahead even if you make it through being a guinea pig for new test drugs and with all the increased awareness. This cancer "journey" I have been on is not like backpacking through Europe or taking a chance on an Airbnb, and it's certainly not an adventure anybody would ever choose to take. Having cancer is a never-ending detour from the good stuff of life, a sojourn through a specific hell that keeps on giving, even when you're "cured." Being diagnosed, treated (in various ways), surviving, and then presenting again, for a full four times in all, and then going through my transplant has impacted every single facet of my life. From the moment you are told you have a malignant tumor to the time you are told you are in remission, you go places, see sides of humanity, and face your own humanity in ways you could never have dreamed. And let me tell you, even when you have been through it before, when it comes around again, you're still going to discover wonderfully horrific new facts that you need to deal with, adapt to, and accept. Yeah, cancer!

Hopefully, when you do indeed come out on the other side, you love life more, appreciate the things you never noticed before, and will come to live that "don't sweat the small stuff" saying nearly every day of your life post-cancer. But things aren't always so rosy in living life. Heck, even without surviving cancer, life can be tough, right?

Not everyone is familiar with or even wants to talk about the dark side of survivorship. It's like having Darth Vader breathing down your neck; you don't want to turn around and face him, but he is always there. The default assumption is often: "They're cured. They're good now." However, privately, many survivors battle a multitude of other prolonged health problems and personal issues: depression, financial trouble, employment issues. And when you're no longer the cute kid with cancer, your hashtag doesn't trend as well on Twitter.

Needless to say, you might end up being more anxious in some ways (which I am, I know), and as you chug along through life, happy to be cancer-free, making plans like you never could before, suddenly something can trigger you—a smell like something you used to smell down a hospital hallway, a song playing on a car radio that you heard almost every day when you drove back and forth to the clinic, the way somebody says their name with a certain tone or timbre in their voice that reminds you of that kid you met so long ago, somebody you haven't seen since those days playing with him in the playroom at a Ronald McDonald House—and then you get to thinking, whatever happened to that kid? Heck, whatever happened to all those kids I saw undergoing the same treatments as me during the four times I had to be treated? You know the likelihood they all survived is slim; the odds don't play out that way in the poker game of life.

See, I could spin my mind round and round and round for days over these kinds of questions. It feels like countless emotions and glimpses of memories set on replay; you see and feel every memory as if it happened yesterday.

Then there are the people I have met who are deeply angry at the cards they were dealt, even if they somehow managed to turn over a winning hand to survive and remain cancer-free. The emotions I'm talking about are well past feeling sorry for yourself. Cancer temporarily takes you out of the game of life, and even if you make it to play another day, you can be mighty pissed off that you got waylaid even for the shortest period, let alone if you are walking around still suffering from the aftereffects of treatment that many cancer survivors are.

Yes, whenever you have cancer, no matter the type and your circumstance, surviving it gives you perspective. And someone like me, who has been through much soul searching to get to a place where I can write this book and proclaim I am currently in remission, "surviving," for want of a better word, is the most critical part of my story.

In the last Rocky movie, *Rocky Balboa*, not that *Creed* one where Rocky played a supporting character (but good old Stallone got an Oscar nomination for it, how about that!), Stallone as "Rocky" says to the actor playing his son, "It ain't about how hard ya hit. It's about how hard you can get hit and keep moving forward. How much you can take and keep moving forward. That's how winning is done!"

This is how I feel. It's less about the fact that I got through all the hardship that I did and more about what I do now, moving forward each day—that's really what matters. And one of those things that I feel is important in moving forward, God knows, is writing this book, and especially coming to this chapter where I let you know all I know about survival. And maybe that will give someone hope that moving forward is the best way to survive.

I Wish I Could Remember All the Things I Have Forgotten and Forget Much of What I Remember

One complication for many of us cancer survivors, something I have mentioned before and certainly something that affects me daily—to a frustrating degree, actually—is my memory loss. Inevitably, almost every cancer patient gets waylaid by "chemo brain," those terribly fuzzy days and nights when your mind is just not working right. But for me, specifically, I have suffered terrible long-term memory loss, so much so that I had to enlist my mom in writing this book to help me cover the gaps I have, or to set me straight about when something happened and with whom it happened. This is my own personal hell, I know, and I suffer through it in silence most of the time, along with other survivors. Sometimes I have trouble finding a particular word, like that one that means, you know, that word that starts with an "S," or is it an "F"? I think—anyway, I forget, get confused, and get frustrated. And this can affect others that I interact with. Sometimes I'm affected in my personal life, or in the line at the coffee shop, or more importantly, at work. I find myself making lists all the time, jotting down notes and reviewing things sometimes to the exhaustion of coworkers and friends. A lousy memory like mine is often seen as a weakness by employers; they don't understand it. I even know of quite a few acquaintances who assumed I had ADD or that I simply didn't care enough to concentrate. I know my bad memory has kept me from getting a job, in some instances. With this type of issue comes a variety of responses, sometimes negative and sometimes rude. But hey, I understand it; my memory loss can be frustrating for everyone.

The cool thing, I guess, is that I can watch the same movie over and over and be just as entertained as the first time around. This always reminds me of that scene in *National Lampoon's European Vacation*. My family watched that movie a lot; my dad was a mad Chevy Chase fan. Anyway, there is a scene in the film where the Griswold family gets stuck in one of those London roundabout traffic circles, and they go round and round for what always struck me (and strikes me still) as a funny gag. As their car circles and circles, Chevy "Clark" Griswold keeps repeating, "Look, kids, Big Ben, Parliament... Big Ben, Parliament." This is the way it is with my memory. I have to be reminded of things over and over to remember them. I indeed have seen *European Vacation* plenty of times, and I laugh anew at this scene every time I see it.

As I get older, I fear my memory problems will get worse. I mean, it's natural to start forgetting stuff as you get older, right? But I wonder, will regular memory loss be doubly problematic for me? I'm already walking around with these great big holes in my memory to begin with. But then again, maybe I am forgetting so many of the details about my chemo treatments, surgeries, and the other bad events about my years of having cancer that this memory loss is, in some ways, as much a blessing as it is a curse. And, as I get older, I fear my memory problems will get worse. (See what I did there? Bad joke? Maybe, but it is the way my life is sometimes. I say something, and already I have forgotten that I said it.)

As far as a blessing, maybe I've been able to forget a large percentage of the stupid things I've both done and said. That would genuinely free up a lot (debatable) of brain space. Or, maybe sometime soon I'll be able to forget about that time I totally missed the urinal while lying in the ER in V-tach. Or hey, I know, maybe I'll forget about that time that doctor let his residents study my private region when I was highly medicated.

My Heart

Of course, a current physical side effect of what I have gone through is that my heart is compromised. Before last year's heart procedure, I found myself in and out of the hospital, or at least running to the doctor (sometimes as much as two times a week) to get my ticker checked. "Look, Big Ben, Parliament... again," like last year when my resting heart rate hit upward of 250 beats per minute—I told you about that in the intro to this book. It's the heart, man; dire stuff.

As you must suspect, I am limited in some of the physical activities I can do. I have to be a little cautious. Makes sense, right? These concerns took me away from practicing martial arts, which was, at one time, so important in my life. But I do other activities now, have made some adjustments—survivors are great adjusters—in finding ways to remain active. I work out by doing a cardio routine, and I also lift weights at the gym. I'm not about to curl up on the couch with a big bag of Fritos and a beer just because I can't do some physical activities. Like anybody, I need to keep fit.

I do have to say, though, that most doctors think I'm surprisingly healthy, given my history and circumstances. I still manage to practice some martial arts, "hit the bag," and have remained a steady weight these past few years, which is an accomplishment for a man whose childhood nicknames included "Skeletor," "No-ass-at-all," etc. It's a cruel world, right?

How I Feel

Emotionally, well, I missed out on much of what one usually gets in a normal childhood. You read that the times I did have with my friends and family were truly fantastic, and they were. But they were always colored by either the fact that I was sick, had just gotten over being sick, or always had, in the back of my mind, the idea that I could be sick again. Is it true that what doesn't kill you makes you stronger? I guess, but whatever it is that you don't die from takes its toll physically, mentally, and certainly emotionally.

Honestly, at times I feel like my body and emotions are "out of sync"; I feel like certain stages of growing up never progressed as they should have naturally. And, because of that, I generally feel a bit "off." But I suck it up, try to appreciate what I have and what I've learned, and get through it. That's certainly what my Granddaddy Hamner would have done.

In a lot of ways, though, certainly when it comes to emotions and my psychological makeup, I'll never truly know what I'm missing. How could I? At almost every step of the way, my life has been interrupted by cancer, its recurrences, and the side effects of treatment. I couldn't develop relationships fully, did not progress as a normal kid my age, could never fully enjoy vacations, college, etc. I have walked through the world (or been pushed in a wheelchair through it) always feeling something was missing.

Maybe for me, at least in this regard, I can best explain it as a "never had it, don't know what I am missing" kind of a thing. I do know for sure that I missed out on some specific aspects of emotional and psychological development that most people get to go through. I believe that my music, being able to write songs and connect with people through my art, helped bridge the emotional disconnect gap. God knows, I met some truly wonderful people when I was singing my songs, whether in bars, out playing for patients in hospitals, or even in dealing with some of the "interesting" characters in the music business. Although I know that I lack in some ways, I also know that my experiences have tested my mind and spirit, offering a way for me to see the opportunity in the difficulties of life. My choice is always to become better rather than bitter.

And, not to get too personal here, but surely my romantic possibilities have been lessened, truncated, and not as explored as well as they could have been had I not been so sick. I have dated a good amount and appreciate all the ladies I have met in my life, be they friends or something a little more. But again, my personal POV has always been colored by my history and how much of those experiences I felt I could share with someone. Some women have been interested, others not so much, and still others could never see the "me" beyond the guy who endured cancer.

Insurance

Not that health care in the US isn't a nightmare pretty much for everybody these days, but should you have a preexisting or chronic condition, possibly in need of what's referred to as "catastrophic care" (or the possibility of it), man, you can find yourself behind the financial eight ball pretty quickly — or facing bankruptcy even.

I'm not about to get political here. I don't know nor care what side you're on politically. This goes beyond all that. If you happen to be rich, what's the worry? You can find and afford excellent health care, the best doctors, and manage any copay and deductibles. Things are pretty good. If you happen to be poor, from my research and in many cases, all you have to do is to prove that you can't afford healthcare, and voilà! You have it. Now, I'm not saying you are going to get the best doctors or care in this scenario, but you won't go broke… not that you could, because, if you're poor, you have no money anyway.

Sure, in both scenarios some people are cheating the system and others are paying into it fairly. And both political sides will give you examples of both the good guys and the bad by usually bragging about themselves or blaming each other about why either exists.

What I am concerned about is the group I fall into—the middle class. The goal posts move all the time for us, and forget it if you happen to have a preexisting condition. Currently, as of 2019, I am paying almost $900 per month for my coverage, which is up 27% from last year, and I can barely afford it. I have no choice. As you have already read, I go in to see doctors, run to hospitals and clinics quite frequently, and the procedures I face are usually quite costly. Years back, I was even denied coverage, and on another occasion, I was considering full-on disability, which I didn't end up taking in the end, as the process there is rather flawed. But, because of what I've outlined here, jobs aren't so easy for me to come by or to keep, so my money situation is sometimes precarious at best.

Believe me, you'll find out really quick that even when you think you have good coverage, you may not have it as good as you need it if you are chronically ill—the very time that someone needs good health coverage. Ironically, though, I believe those who are the most at risk are people who have some big health dilemma happen to them but are not chronically ill. At least I've been through the process enough times to know about what could be out there when it comes to health coverage — good and not so great.

The Dreaded Job Search

A good part of what I struggle with most these days is trying to find a job. I think this is probably true for anybody who has gone through something life threatening or is still facing health challenges. It's not that I go to an interview wearing a "Hey, I have been up to bat with Hodgkin's lymphoma four times" badge, but the trials and tribulations of my health history are part of my life. And more and more, I see how they affect my job prospects.

While I won't avoid talking about the challenges cancer has thrown my way, once a possible employer gets ahold of that fact about my life, some can't help *but* talk about it... not that it's legal to ask questions about my health history when interviewing me. Still, they do. Sure, it is better now than it used to be. There is less stigma around having had cancer, but once you have had it, sometimes the world will always consider cancer first... then you. I hate to say this, but all of us who have survived are lepers in a way, too often defined by the disease.

It's amazing, actually. Some of these companies play their cancer card in a slick way. At certain times of the year, they hold "raise money for cancer" walks, and then say: "Hey, look what good we did for cancer research, patients, and survivors." However, when it comes down to hiring those who have beat the disease or those who are struggling afterward from it, many of these companies don't "talk their walk." Too many of them are skittish about hiring cancer survivors, or they hold to an unspoken policy of not hiring anyone who has ever been chronically ill. Sure, it's hypocritical, but I think this is all just people scared of those things they fear most in life... and want to never think about.

Look, I'm not saying my particular survivor challenges—failing memory, having to leave for doctor's appointments, those days I am completely fatigued—do not impinge on my productivity. But I can guarantee you that I'm motivated to work—like so many other survivors—and I'll be sure to make up the time I lose. I'm always down for whatever challenge is presented. Most cancer survivors know they are managing an uphill climb out there in the workforce. I think you'll find, because of what we have been through and because we have to prove ourselves time and again, that we are some of the hardest workers out there.

Caregivers

Whole books have been written on and about caregivers of the chronically ill. Friends, spouses, parents, kids—a caregiver can come in any shape or size, from anyplace in your life, and be on hand a day, a year, months, maybe just the occasional phone call. For my purposes, I am not talking about medical staff (a whole other level of caregiver and amazing people, to be sure), and I am not talking here about a person who you only see from time to time; they are essential too, to be sure. What I am writing about in this section is the full-time caregiver, someone who is around all the time, administering love, support, medicine, etc. Someone you know that you could not have survived without.

For me, as you know, that person is my mom. For the many reasons I give in this book, and many more you can assume, plus the many I could never articulate let alone write, my mom is the person I think of first and foremost as my caregiver. This is also another part of the book where I have my mom weigh in. I think it is equally important for a caregiver to have a say, especially a parent who has been a caregiver. My mom's perspective—what she has come to think about all of my battles and treatments now so many years after the fact, how she views life presently, what her conclusions are as she lives each day as a caregiver of a survivor—is an integral part of the overall picture, I feel. She has been in the trenches with me all the way, and if you have someone in your life who has done the same for you, or you are that someone who never truly knew where to turn when things were at their bleakest for the cancer patient you were caring for, or if you are even now consoling and counseling other caregivers (cancer is everywhere, man; the odds are too good on this), my mom's POV here will be a comfort.

Incredible as it is to understand, Ryan—as sick as he has been—has always been my support. Sure, there have been family members and friends, phenomenal doctors and nurses. But, no one else in the world has "been there" with a smile, a thumbs-up, an "okay, just tell me what to do" in the middle of our "war." Once, when Ryan was going through the bone marrow transplant, he and I woke up in the hospital room to blood—lots of blood—covering one side of his bed from an IV gone askew. I jumped from my fold-out-up-and-over hospital chair and quickly got the nurse's attention to take care of our early morning nightmare. Soon, things were back on track—no sign of that awful vision with imagination over the edge—and I remember, as usual, Ryan making a joke to make his nurse laugh before leaving the room. Afterward, we sat silent for a few minutes, me thanking God for His care, Ryan thoughtful before speaking to me. Again, speaking words I can never forget, words I hold onto, Ryan said, "Mom, wouldn't it be great—after all this is over—if you are strong like you are now, and Dad can relax." Yes, I thought, that would be wonderful. And, the wonder was in the insight Ryan had given to me at that moment.

Years later, as a young adult, Ryan lived in the small summer house at the back of my property. He lived there for two years before taking a corporate job and moving out of state. But, in those two years, we would borrow from Charles Dickens, "It was the best of times; it was the worst of times," as it truly was. Within those two years, Ryan completed his "Hear the Heart" tour of the Southeast, visiting children's clinics and hospitals, performing his music, and speaking to those who needed the encouragement of someone who had been where they were. He would compose his cottage tunes, right there in an actual cottage, and I had the privilege of experiencing Ryan's talent of putting his heart into words and recording the music that inspires others today. I want to imagine a hundred years from now a historical plaque mounted at the front door of his cottage that reads, "Ryan Hamner, maker of words, lover of coffee, singer, writer, musician, survivor—lived here once, writing his 'cottage tunes,' inspiring thousands, but mostly his mom."

We lived for a while with me teaching school and Ryan working his business online, selling hats and miscellany found mostly at yard sales, estate sales, and antique shops. I can remember boxing the hats and helping him load them into the back of his car to take to the post office. He built an income for himself and while he was employed in this endeavor, which partially supported his music and his "Hear the Heart" tour, one of the most enjoyable things we did was to ramble through local yard sales on Saturday mornings. He'd find collectibles, like vintage ashtrays I'd never recognize, and he'd sell them for great profit. We developed a challenge to find the most unique ashtray. And one day, browsing through a local antique shop, I picked up an ashtray from the 40s. On the front was a 3D image of a woman in a bathing suit, one arm over her tilted head showing off her 3D breasts. I handed it to Ryan, as I believed I had won our contest and found the most unique ashtray. He turned it over to reveal the bottom of the ashtray with the 3D image of the backside of the woman. We laughed, I won, and Ryan sold it for profit. I miss that ashtray, but the memory is priceless.

As this business dissolved, money was tight. Ryan collected rejection notices from job applications along with letters from insurance companies turning him down because of his preexisting condition. We still dealt with his health issues, sending him to the ER in town and several times to Emory in Atlanta. My teaching career was coming to a close as I was planning to retire from the classroom with half the years in that most teachers are able to invest. Teaching school for me had been difficult, taking leaves of absence when necessary to help Ryan. During this time, I was a little more stressed than usual, coming home every now and then with a bad "teacher attitude." One day, as I got home and walked through the back door, I found Ryan working at my computer, probably applying for more jobs. For me, he was conveniently sitting within earshot, and I had had a day filled with disrespectful students and difficult administration. Listening for a minute, Ryan calmly turned around, smiled at me, threw a crumpled wad of paper, and said something so ridiculous that I had to laugh and get over the little things that had stressed me out that day, helping me remember that at that moment neither one of us was dealing with any of those usual major things we had dealt with in the past. Ryan wasn't in ICU; I wasn't sleeping in the fold-down-up-and-around hospital chair and waiting for news from the doctor. Right then, we were okay. We were experiencing a time that will never come again. It was a good day.

And so, we learned to appreciate the good times that make up just a moment sometimes, a day maybe, sometimes a week or two, and maybe a few months that have not involved an emergency, a procedure, a time of fear and exhaustion.

Memories, for me, come like patchwork, edges frayed at times. But, the good ones put together, become what we hold onto, even the smallest moment can mean the greatest joy. Sometimes, in the mornings, during Ryan's "cottage years" with me, he'd make breakfast for both of us up at the big house. His favorite, I think, was fresh blueberry protein pancakes. One morning, as he mixed and poured the batter onto the hot griddle, I stood watching and talking about something insignificant. He asked if I'd like blueberries in my pancakes as he dropped the fresh berries onto his pancakes. "Of course," I said, admiring his cooking expertise. Without a grin, he dropped a berry onto my pancake, stopped, admired his creation, and dropped another. Putting the berries down and flipping his pancakes loaded with blueberries, he looked up at me and grinned, making me laugh and now remember.

That was a time I'll always have, boxing hats, eating blueberry pancakes, listening to music in its creation, and learning over and again what is important. For Ryan, music has always been essential. It's part of who he is. He told me once, "Mom, I'll always be playing my guitar and singing. That's just who I am." And then, just a few years ago, I learned by accident that Ryan had sold his guitar. I was shocked and asked him why he would sell the instrument he loved. "Mom," he said, "I'll get a better one later. Don't worry. I had to sell it to get the airline tickets to fly to Cleveland." I knew he had a doctor's appointment there; I just didn't know he was so short of funds to get there. Ryan knew I would have done whatever I needed to do to keep him from selling his guitar; he just wanted to handle it on his own—would never have asked me for the money. That's just who he is. That was his part of taking care of me.

But, this was not so different in better times, when finances were not so tight. Once, I accompanied Ryan to a car dealership when he was planning to trade in his car. He knew that I had been "trading in" my thirteen-year-old Honda Accord—one part at a time. That day, Ryan found a car for me, negotiated the deal, and paid the down payment so I would be safe on the road.

Sometimes, the "best of times" happens in the "worst of times"—in spite of them, and maybe, because of them. All I know for certain is that I have experienced fresh blueberries in protein pancakes, a wad of paper thrown with a smile, "cottage tunes," hats in boxes, and a reversible ashtray with boobs. Those things I'd never change, never trade.

I let Mom interject without censoring her here, as I did everywhere. But reading the above, I kinda got choked up. The things she remembers: blueberry pancakes, that ashtray, my eBay business, all that stuff I do happen to remember. But what gets me most is when my mom writes how I was her support. Well, back at ya, Mom, one hundred times over and around back again.

See, that's the thing with surviving. Sure, there are all those challenges I mentioned above. They are real and they get in my way, as they get in the way of all of us who have or have had cancer. But there's life-changing, human-spirit empowering stuff that comes out of this battle. Caregivers and patients, the true survivors, affect one another's lives in ways we never can imagine. I mean, it's obvious to even those who have, thankfully, never gone through what my mom and I have been through, how those who care for you do indeed become so important in your life. But what is less obvious is the courage/strength and inspirations cancer survivors reveal in such little ways and how we can come to inspire each other as well as those who are not sick. I guess that's what my mom means by me being her support, but God knows I never look at myself that way. As far as I am concerned, it was always me leaning on her. But as I felt when writing my children's cancer book and singing my songs on tour, as I feel right now, writing this chapter on survival, lots of life-affirming stuff comes out of a story like mine—people, places, and circumstances that I have affected positively. And man, if that doesn't give you hope…

Chapter 8

The Choice of Perspective:
What Do You See?

If something, an affliction, happens to you, you either let it defeat you, or you defeat it.

–Jean-Jacques Rousseau

Before I hit you with this book's ending, something I think is really important and uplifting (yeah, and heavy), I wanted to tell you this humorous story about my cousin Justin breaking me out of the hospital for the day and him getting pulled over. To be specific, I was allowed to get out for the day, but I was weak, recovering from my bone marrow transplant. And my cousin taking me for a ride, as much as us getting pulled over, was the most excitement I had experienced in a long time.

I felt like he had truly broken me out of jail for the day, and I was so happy to be free. The transplant had definitely messed up my entire system, and my body was never able to warm up naturally for a long while afterward. But that didn't deter my enthusiasm for getting away. I simply bundled up in layers, wearing my hooded sweatshirt and the toboggan I was used to wearing in the hospital.

And then, not more than half an hour out, we got pulled over, again with my cousin driving, the cop giving us those terse and tension-filled instructions from behind my cousin's car: "Driver, out of the car. Show me your hands and keep walking backward, slowly." Wow! Were we being punk'd? Had we driven through an episode of *Live PD*? I simply sat as still as I could in the passenger's seat, cold—I had gone through my bone marrow transplant two weeks before—and on top of that, now I had a bad case of nerves.

I was so happy to be broken out of the hospital that day. I was as glad to see my cousin as I was to be taken for a ride like a happy puppy in the front seat. I had been lying in my hospital bed staring out the window of Emory University Hospital, aching to get out, walk among people, step down sidewalks, slip in and out of buildings, drive in a car—simply to get into the hustle and bustle of a normal day. I so missed normal. People really do take their everyday freedoms for granted, I thought, and when my cousin Justin came to get me I knew, despite how weak I felt, I wouldn't waste a moment of my release that day. Sure, I had to return to my hospital room all too soon, but being out for even a short time was an amazing feeling I'll never forget.

But here we were being pulled over by the police. I hadn't given much thought to how I was dressed when leaving the hospital, but as I mentioned, I was cold because I was recovering from the massive procedure I had just gone through. On that afternoon, a mild September day in Atlanta, the hooded sweatshirt paired with the germ mask I had to wear definitely made a statement. Yes, not too many people get cold in September in Atlanta, certainly not so cold to be bundled up as I was (nor are most Atlanteans usually seen wearing surgical masks), but hey man, I had just gone through a bone marrow transplant. Give me a break, OK?

But I also needed to give the cop a break. Most times, a police officer coming upon one guy out driving another guy, with the passenger dressed like me (really, imagine how I looked!), he'd probably be stopping the commission of a crime. My cousin and I had to have been an interesting pair, to say the least.

Everything came out OK in the end. No harm, no foul. The policeman listened long and hard to my cousin, and he assessed that we weren't what he thought we were... although what we were he probably had no idea, even after my cousin explained. He let us go without even a warning, and my cousin tooled us around for another hour or so, with me just enjoying the sun on my face and smelling the fresh air... and no more stops by the cops. To this day I still get a chuckle over thinking of those first few thoughts that had to have passed through that policeman's mind that day when he saw us. See, sometimes the result of cancer and its treatment can make life kind of fun.

OK, now on with the heavy stuff...

I have struggled writing this book trying to remember some details, wanting not to remember others, trying to put in clear and concise language all that happened to me during my cancer journey, during my life. But now I find I come to what, for me, is turning out to be the hardest part of this book to write. I wanted to end this all with a specific idea of what the journey has brought me to and where I hope I am going.

I don't say this next statement aloud very often, if I ever have at all, but I do think it a lot: Some of the best opportunities in my life have come out of this awful disease I had... and had... and had... and had. I know I kind of danced around that idea in the pages above, and you are probably saying: "Ryan, are you nuts? What possible opportunities came from being diagnosed four times with cancer, suffering through all the treatments, being plucked over and over from a normal growing up?"

Besides the unique journey my life has taken and being left with a whole bunch of experiences not many folks have had (yeah, I am a helluva lot of fun at parties, I can tell you that) maybe, just maybe, I appreciate each day a bit more than the guy or girl next door. I told you previously that sometimes you come out of experiences such as I've had hating the world, scolding God with a "Why me?" all the time. Or you could come out of experiences like mine just darn glad that you survived. There's a wide chasm between these perspectives, but there it is: ***perspective.***

I used to think that life was like a beach (yes, I said beach, with an "e" and an "a"). The way I imagined it was that we all had a certain amount of sand we got to lay out on over our lifetime. The ocean waves came in and out, pulling that sand away (in the challenges we faced) as much as washing in some gems (friends, family, love, professional accomplishments). The way I saw it, we all had a finite amount of that sand, and sooner or later, even if you lived to be ninety, your beach completely eroded by the slow passage of the tides of time.

But these days, despite how much erosion I have felt in my life, I imagine my beach stretching to the horizon. I know it ends; it has to. All of our life "property" ends (build as many condos and Tiki huts as you like, you can't take them with you). But from the current clear place where I am, the way I look at life now, or more precisely the *choice* I *make* on what *perspective* I *take*, I feel an infinite horizon of sand at my back, as I do limitless clear blue water ahead.

OK, enough of the metaphor now. What I am trying to say here is, despite what you have read of my journey, regardless of all the obstacles I have faced and will always face in surviving, I do feel pretty light in my step. Why?

Well, like I just wrote, it's *the choice I make on what perspective I take*.

I know there are days you do not want to get out of bed, especially if that bed is in a hospital. There are those days you are wondering if the treatments you are undergoing will make you as sick as they did the last time. Days when you worry about what you are putting your family through as much as what you're putting your body, mind, and spirit through. I know how fear can grab you so hard, the only way to even get through the next few minutes is to imagine that what's happening to you is a movie you are watching and not what you are enduring in your life.

I have been there, I know. But as sure as I struggled my way puking up my guts, was nearly smothered by smells I will go to my grave never forgetting and will do anything never to smell again, as much as I am happy that some of my memory is burned to ash and at the same time I am pissed that it is, I can tell you with complete assurance that the ability we all have—and I think should use as often as we can, no matter what's coming at us—is the ability to change how we look at things. How we come to . . .

Choose the Right Perspective

Through all my years dealing with cancer, I never could change a diagnosis (man, how nice would that be, right?). The side effects came at me as a result of my treatments based on my doctors' opinions. Like many others before me and too many to follow, I just had to get through what I had to get through, in my fashion, and get on with getting on... even during those times I felt I couldn't go on. But the one thing I learned, the thing that I could change and did change over and over again (even through the process of writing this book I changed it) is my perspective.

I, Ryan Hamner, yes *that* Ryan Hamner, your tour guide through the last eight chapters here, can choose how I see things. And deciding how I look at things ultimately determines how I feel... about those things, and how they will or will not impact my life. This choice isn't always so easy. Faced with seemingly insurmountable hurdles or life-threatening circumstances, entertaining various choices can be quite a challenge, let alone making decisions. The last thing I was seeing were the choices laid out before me during those days I couldn't even lift my head from my sweaty, bad-smelling pillow. But a change in perspective is available to all of us all the time.

When you're young and sick, your world seems black and white. A kid feeling pain, sickness, fear, and anxiety tends to concentrate on the time when all those bad feelings will depart from his or her life; this kid has a limited view with few choices in perspective. And believe me, especially when you're young and sick or your disease rolls over into something chronic, it's so easy to become conditioned to live in fear. You are always waiting for that next sudden blast in your ear, right when you've gotten comfortable in bed and are falling to sleep. You walk around jittery 24/7, suspecting some awful monster of a circumstance to come around the corner every time you let your guard down for even a short afternoon when you're successfully able to distract yourself enough with some activity to forget your cancer for an hour. Or you experience some side effect or a new treatment that you didn't hear or understand when the doctors explained it to you. Surprise, surprise!

When you're older, you have the ability to look back and realize that so much of your life was stolen because of your illness. You have heard that saying: "You can't go home again," right? Well, I got one that's even better: "Your past can come to steal your future." And although nobody wants this, it does happen to many people (me included), and because of that thievery, you come to fear the future. Things like love, relationships—every facet of life, actually—is colored by the terrible stuff in one's past, and like everybody else, you are a product of that past, but a cancer survivor's past is some deep muddy stuff, man!

But I am living proof (if there's such a thing as "dead proof"; I never hear anybody use that phrase… sorry, I digress) that even with all of that nasty stuff messing up your past, stealing your thunder, making it hard to deal with life in the here and now, you can come out on the other side with a choice on how you view life.

I choose not to see days of being sick and having to be picked up from school because I was so nauseous from harsh chemo treatments. I decide instead to see my days back then leaving school on a beautiful sunny afternoon and burning down the road in a Corvette with the badass granddaddy I adored. I don't want to focus on that day, as a sixth grader, when I was diagnosed with cancer for the third time; I want to focus on going to the skateboard shop right after we got the news and building my dream skateboard. Life is an ever-changing collage of feelings, and by choosing the right perspectives, I think we can help cover the painful feelings with better ones. Yes, the old stuff will always be underneath, but the new picture will be what we see, live, and feel.

It ultimately comes down to you asking yourself what thoughts you want to breathe life into: your actual memories of struggles, pain, fear, and anxiety, or what you learned from those struggles and the "good" threaded throughout those hard times. Which will you choose to see as defeated? You, or your disease?

Made in the USA
Columbia, SC
18 May 2019